The Situ Test

BMA

Edited by

Michael Stoddart

Robbie Ley Greaves

© 2018 MD+ Publishing

Published by: MD+ Publishing

Cover Design: Alexander Logan

ISBN-10: 0995662622

ISBN-13: 978-0995662629

Printed in the United Kingdom

CONTENTS

Acknowledgements

Written and Edited by Mr Michael Stoddart and Dr Robbie Ley Greaves.

We owe great thanks to all those listed below who worked hard to contribute questions to the book and whose help has been invaluable.

Dr Conrad Harrison
Dr Odhran Keating
Dr George Hill
Dr Laura Wilkinson
Dr John Shenouda
Dr Heather Stirling
Dr Harry Posner

Thank you for purchasing the book and we hope you find it helpful in preparing for the exam.

Michael and Robbie

INTRO

1 INTRO

1 | Introduction

What is the Situational Judgement Test (SJT)?

When applying to the UK Foundation Programme, final year medical students are ranked nationally based on their:

Educational Performance Measure (50 points) – up to 43 points depending on their decile within their own medical school, with an additional 7 points available for extra degrees and publications.

Situational Judgement Test (50 points) – run twice a year (December and January depending on medical school), this is a multiple-choice examination designed to test 'the professional attributes expected of the Foundation Doctor'. The paper is marked and once both tests are done, translated into a 0-50 scale. This is done based on the distribution of EPM score for that year.

It is therefore important to note that the SJT makes up 50% of an applicant's total score, and so being familiar with the style of questions and subject matter is key.

What are the different question types?

The SJT contains 70 different questions, each with a clinical scenario. Of the 70 individual questions, only 60 will be counted, the remaining 10 will be used for future exams. The questions are divided into two different types, ranking questions (40) and multiple-choice questions (20). Each ranking question is marked out of 20, and each multiple-choice question is marked out of 12

Ranking questions – these questions ask students to rank the available answers (A-E) in order of most appropriateness (1-5). Full marks are scored by correctly ranking each answer.

Multiple choice questions – these questions give 8 possible answers and students are to pick 3. There is no ranking for these questions, each correct answer is worth 4 marks, giving a maximum of 12.

What content will be covered?

The SJT is designed to test 'the professional attributes expected of the Foundation Doctor'. It is important for students to judge each situation as if they were a Foundation Year 1 (F1) doctor. There is no syllabus as such and so 'revision' can be daunting, however the official SJT guidance, person specification, and importantly the GMC Good Medical Practice guides are good places to start. The UKFPO website states the questions will focus on five professional attributes:

1)   Commitment to professionalism
2)   Coping with pressure
3)   Effective communication
4)   Patient focus
5)   Working effectively as part of a team.

We also recommend students clarify certain aspects of the Foundation Programme including; clinical/educational supervisors, consenting for procedures, FP10 prescriptions and discharging patients.

2 | TIPS

TIPS

2 | Tips For Answering Questions

There is no fool-proof system to answering the SJT. The official advice is that this exam cannot be revised for, however, understanding how the paper is marked will prevent time from being wasted, and so give students the best chance of scoring well.

Students have 140 minutes to complete the SJT in invigilated exam conditions. This equates to 2 minutes per question. This is a short amount of time to read the scenario, 'judge', and fill in the computer mark sheet. There is a real risk that students run out of time, and fail to complete the paper. Any questions left blank will score zero, this could potential have a huge effect on the final SJT score as we will discuss later. We therefore recommend strictly sticking to the 2 minute per question timing, and most importantly ensure that all questions on the mark sheet are completed, even if it is guesswork!

Ranking style questions

As described above, the ranking questions are scored out of 20, so for each of the 5 responses one can score 4 marks. This mark reduces depending on how far the student has ranked the answer from the 'true' position. This can be shown in the table below:

Ideal Rank	Student Rank 1	Student Rank 2	Student Rank 3	Student Rank 4	Student Rank 5
D	4	3	2	1	0
C	3	4	3	2	1
E	2	3	4	3	2
A	1	2	3	4	3
B	0	1	2	3	4

Giving different responses the same rank will score both 0. The minimum score available per completed question is 8/20. A guess will on average score 14/20.

We recommend, given the short time limit and pressure to complete the paper, students should concentrate on ranking the best and worst responses first. Then if time allows consider ranking the middle 3, however even if this is guessed, achieving the best and worst answers will give a minimum of 16/20.

Multiple choice style questions

These differ from the ranking questions, as only the 3 correct answers are marked, meaning there is a possibility of scoring 0/12. Because of this, some students opt to do these questions before the ranking style, allowing them the opportunity to 'guess' the remaining ranking questions if they run out of time – this would give an average of 14/20, with a minimum of 8/20 for a completed

TIPS

answer. Compare that with 0/12 for either leaving blank or incorrectly answering an MCQ, or 0/20 for leaving a ranking question blank.

Selecting more than 3 responses will result in a score of 0 for the whole question.

Marking

As described previously, of the 70 questions included in each paper, only 60 are "live". The score that each student receives is scaled from 0 to 50, with the distribution of the scores set to match the mean and distribution of the EPM scores for that cohort. This is to try to give both the EPM and SJT scores equal weighting for the applicant.

An equation is used to turn the raw SJT score into the scaled score. For the 2017 cohort it was as follows:

Scaled SJT Score = Equated Raw SJT Score x 0.132 – 76.742

This will change from year to year, but will provide a useful estimate of potential scores when using the mock in this book.

Importantly, the distribution of scores an almost normal distribution. This means that in the 2017 SJT 95% of candidates were within 2 standard deviations of the mean. With such a small standard deviation, and so narrow distribution, missing or scoring zero on some questions can have a dramatic impact on the final scaled SJT mark awarded.

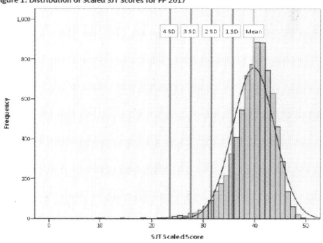

Figure 1: Distribution of Scaled SJT Scores for FP 2017

Mean: 39.78
Median: 40.30
Standard Deviation: 4.07

Finally

There is are two true mock tests available through the FPAS website, the questions and answers in this book are only used as a guide of topics and question types.

Familiarise yourself with a copy of the mark sheet, which is available on the FPAS website. As you will be unlikely to go back through the paper given the limited time available, make sure that all questions are filled in i.e. each ranking question has five different ranks, and the multiple choice questions have three different choices.

We recommend using these official mocks in the weeks running up the exam under timed conditions and importantly, using the mark sheet in order to get used to filling in the answers.

TIPS

3 Foundation Doctor Roles and Responsibilities

ROLES

3   Foundation Doctor Roles and Responsibilities

As previously mentioned, when answering the SJT it is important you assume the role of a Foundation Year 1 doctor. By clarifying some of these roles, we hope not only you are able to answer the questions more effectively, but also have a head start when you start working.

Training

Your foundation years are as part of a recognised training programme, and so as part of continuing professional development you are required to record evidence of this, as well as working towards training goals as set out at your educational and clinical supervisor meetings.

Clinical supervisors: are often one of the consultants you directly work for, and will change with each rotation. They are responsible for your clinical progress during your rotation in their department and will compile a report at the end. They will be your first port of call with clinical issues in the department during your rotation.

Educational supervisors: will stay the same for the entire year. They ensure you set and meet your educational goals, and will meet you at the beginning and end of each placement. They may not directly work with you, however will be involved in recommending your end of year sign off at ARCP. You may need to contact them about training or professional concerns during the Foundation Programme. Each hospital also has a Foundation Programme Director who will oversee the quality of the programme locally.

(For more information please see the FP Reference guide 2016: http://www.foundationprogramme.nhs.uk/download.asp?file=FP_Reference_Guide_2016_-_June_2017_Publication.pdf)

e-Porfolio/Horus: is an electronic log of learning and achievements. There are different work based assessments that need to be completed, and linked to the Foundation Curriculum, during the course of the year to ensure that you are signed off. Reflections can be recorded, and a Team Assessment of Behaviour gives feedback from the multidisciplinary team.

Paperwork

Accurate medical note keeping is an essential skill, and forms part of the legal permanent records. It allows communication between teams, and review can form part of route cause analysis following adverse events. They must include date and time, as well as name and contact number/bleep.

Sick notes: can be issued to cover a period in hospital and where the patient is deemed unfit to work. They can also recommend changes are made to duties to

ROLES

allow the patient to work. They need to remain confidential and so should not go into specifics about individual cases. Patients are able to self certify for up to 1 week without a sick note.

Travel/insurance forms: are generally dealt with by the consultant under whom the patient was admitted under.

Incident forms: are used to document any adverse event or near miss and allow further investigation in order to prevent recurrence. These are often online forms found on the trust intranet, and all healthcare workers have a duty to complete them.

Prescribing: must be safe and accurate, and in line with local/national guidance. You must be aware of allergies and past medical history as you are responsible for the prescriptions you write. F1s cannot write private or community prescriptions (FP10s), nor should they prescribe or administer cytotoxic or immunosuppressant drugs (exception being corticosteroids).

F1s cannot independently discharge patients: They need to be deemed medically fit for discharge (MFFD) by a senior member of the team.

ROLES

4 COMMON TOPICS

TOPICS

4 | Common Topics in SJT Questions

The SJT assumes that candidate has some knowledge of the job of an F1 doctor, and the questions are designed to be answered as such. Answers need to reflect what 'should' be done in each scenario, not necessarily what one 'would' do.

Questions will cover topics as outlined by the GMC's "Duty of a Doctor", as well as the "Person Specification" which can be found on the Foundation Programme website.

Commitment to professionalism:
Appreciating the patient-doctor relationship, and acting with integrity at all times. This includes interactions with colleagues and other healthcare professionals as well as patients. Recognising risks to patient safety, and acting on them.

Coping with pressure:
Ability to manage under pressure, and develop appropriate coping strategies. Recognition of personal emotional and physical well-being, as well as effective time management.

Effective communication:
Able to communicate appropriately with patients and colleagues, using verbal and non-verbal techniques. Ensures understanding and documents thoroughly.

Patient focus:
Acts as the patient's advocate and keeps them at the centre of their care. Acts empathetically and remains professional in the patient-doctor relationship. Ensures confidentially.

Working effectively as part of a team:
Appreciates role in multidisciplinary team in order to provide patient centred care. Understands own self-limitations and where help is available. Offers support to colleagues.

Familiarise yourself with the domains found in the GMC's "Good Medical Practice";

1)   Knowledge, skills and performance
2)   Safety and quality
3)   Communication, partnership and teamwork
4)   Maintaining trust

TOPICS

4.1   Patient safety

A very common topic highlights the need to ensure patient safety at all times. This is covered in the GMC's "Good Medical Practice" and so you must take action if this occurs or is threatened. If this is out of your experience or competence then senior help must be sought.

When an error has occurred the GMC states "You must act immediately to put matters right". Then you must offer an apology and explain fully to the patient what has happened.

1. You are the surgical FY1 on call and are clerking in a patient. You notice that the patients drug chart is already filled out and there are stat orders for IV benzylpenicillin and doxycycline written up to treat a chest infection, which have already been given. There is a medical patient in the bed next door who has been admitted for a chest infection but his drug chart is empty. Neither patient is allergic to anything and all observations are normal. What three things should you do first?

a.   Apologize to the patient
b.   Do nothing as there was no reaction
c.   Re write your patients drug chart
d.   Re write the other patients drug chart
e.   Call the medical FY1 and tell them what has happened
f.   Ask the medical FY1 to apologize to the patient
g.   Complete an incident reporting form
h.   Tell the Medical FY1s clinical supervisor

Answers: A, C, E

Eliminate clearly wrong: B, D, H
Doing nothing does not deal with any possible cause, there is no point rewriting a drug chart already stated to be empty. Nor is contacting their supervisor helpful at the current time.

Reasoning: A – the patient needs to be told and apologized to, this should also be done by the medical FY1 but needs to be done first. C – the patients drug chart needs to be rewritten in order to remove the wrongly written drugs and stop any further drug errors. E – the person who made the error needs to know in the first instance before reporting to anyone else.

2. You are the F1 responsible for weekend ward cover of the cardiology ward. Your responsibilities include a ward round with the on-call cardiology consultant in the morning, they see all the new admissions and unwell patients. You finish the Saturday ward round and the consultant goes home. You then begin seeing the other patients. Later that afternoon you notice there were a number

of new admissions that were not seen by the consultant.

a.   See the new admissions by yourself
b.   Ask the medical registrar to see the new admissions
c.   Call the consultant on call through switchboard, and ask that they come back in to see the patients
d.   See the patients then telephone the consultant on call for advice about their management
e.   See the new admissions yourself today & ask the consultant to see them on the ward round tomorrow.

Best Answer: C
This puts patient care first and rightly informs the consultant that they have been missed.
Worst Answer: A
These are specialist and/or sick cardiology patients, despite your best efforts they should be seen by a consultant and without that their care will be compromised.
Middle answers: D, B, E

Patient safety is the upmost concern here. If these patients have been admitted to an acute cardiology ward, it is usually because they require a specialist cardiology opinion and/or treatment. Therefore C is the safest option. If the consultant is unwilling or unable to return to the ward, asking for advice once you have reviewed the patients is the next best option (D).
Asking the medical registrar to see the patients (B) ensures patient safety, but is a pretty poor allocation of resources, as they will likely have many other unwell and new patients to see. However it would certainly be appropriate for them to review any very unwell patients not seen by the consultant.
The two worst options are to see the patients by yourself without any senior support, though at least with option E they would have a senior review the next day.

4.2   Working with colleagues

Although maintaining good working relationships is important, patient safety must come first. If problems arise there are set protocols with raising concerns with seniors. This is covered in the GMC's "Good Medical Practice", and must be done without delay.
This can be done sensitively, as long a patient safety is not compromised.

3. You are having difficulty with one of your F1 colleagues. One of your peers reports they have been speaking negatively about you in the mess. On ward rounds they frequently attempt to point out your mistakes in front of the consultant.

a.   Confront your colleague directly during the next ward round
b.   Try to correct some of their errors in front of the consultant

c.   Speak directly to their educational supervisor
d.   Speak to the colleague involved in private one afternoon
e.   Speak to your educational supervisor about the colleague

Best Answer: D
Dealing with the issue politely but head on solves it rapidly and reveal any truth in it.
Worst Answer: B
This is petty and does nothing to solve the issue.
Answers: E, C, A

This a very difficult situation, and clearly your colleague is not acting professionally, whatever their reasons for doing so are. If you have issues with a specific person, it is most sensible to speak with them directly about it first (D), though this is best done in a non-confrontational fashion, in private. It is then probably best to speak to your own educational supervisor (E) for advice before speaking to theirs (C).Options A & B are fairly inflammatory, though A is slightly preferable as at least it addresses the issues at hand, rather than combating them with further passive aggression.

4. You are the F1 on an orthopaedic surgery firm. You overhear the consultant making sexist jokes about one of the registrars. During the ward round he makes a sexist remark towards her in your presence. Over the next week he continues to undermine her and asks her to review patients on the ward when she should be with him in theatre. She is clearly upset by the situation.

Rank the following responses in order from most appropriate to least appropriate.

a.   Confront the consultant and tell him you do not think his behaviour is appropriate.
b.   Ask your educational supervisor for advice
c.   Take the registrar for coffee and offer to talk about her situation. Advise her to speak with her Educational supervisor and the Human Resources department.
d.   Report your consultant to the clinical director behind his back.
e.   Do not get involved

Best answer: c
Addressing the situation with the affected person is usually the best answer in these SJT situations
Worst answer: e
Ignoring the problem is invariably the worst answer in the exam
Middle answers: b, d, a
The most appropriate answer is (c), offering to talk about her situation will improve your relationship with her and her educational supervisor and the Human Resources department will be familiar with local protocols regarding bullying and harassment. The least appropriate answer is (e) as you are obliged to oppose

bullying in the workplace. If in doubt you should talk to your educational supervisor (b). Answers

5. You are the SHO in Cardiology and you are approached by one of your female patients who mentions that she was seen by one of your male colleagues last week and that he performed a breast examination on her. After looking in the notes, you do not see any mention of this examination, nor any reasonable indication as to why a breast examination is required.

Rank the following responses in order from most appropriate to least appropriate.

a.   Inform patient advice liaison service
b.   Approach your colleague who conducted the breast examination on your female patient to gain more information regarding this situation
c.   Inform your colleague's clinical supervisor
d.   Report your colleague to the GMC
e.   Document your conversation with the patient in the notes

Best answer: b
This question brings up the issue of a doctor's respect for a patient, which is clearly outlined as an imperative in the GMC's guidance on 'Good Medical Practice'. Considering that you have not been given much information regarding the matter it is best to find out more detail from the colleague, as there may have been a valid reason for the examination.

Worst answer: d
Reporting someone to the GMC is a major step and one that should not be taken lightly, especially without gathering all the relevant information, and may lead to an unwarranted fitness to practice issue.

Middle answers: c, e, a
It would also be prudent to inform a senior member of staff early (C), given that this matter may be exploitation, as someone senior would be better suited to continuing the further investigation. It is always good practice to document conversations with the patient's in the notes (E), but this will not actively help the current situation and is therefore less appropriate than informing a senior member of staff. Informing patient liaison service may help with any complaint in the future but will not be beneficial in the immediate instance.

4.3   Confidentiality

'Maintain and protect patients' information' is one of the core ethical principles for doctors as set by the GMC. The right to confidentiality is paramount in the doctor-patient relationship. There is also a legal duty to keep patient information confidential under the Data Protection Act 1998. A breach of confidentiality can lead to a doctor's fitness to practise to be impaired and can lead to formal review by the GMC.

Despite this there are occasions when confidentiality can be breached. This could be to protect the patient (e.g. sharing information with other HCP regarding treatment), or to protect a member of the public.

Divulging information as required by law – this may be through a court order, even if it is against the patients wishes.

Releasing information for the sake of public interest and safety. This could include treating a neglected child or a vulnerable adult.

These cases where confidentiality needs to be breached without the patients consent should be dealt sensitively, with advice from senior colleagues or indemnity providers.

6. You are an F2 in the Emergency Department. A man has been brought in by paramedics after driving his car into the tree. At the time a passenger in the car mentioned to the paramedic that he thought the driver had had a seizure at the wheel before losing control of the car. The passenger declined to come to hospital and did not leave his contact details. The patient (the driver) works as a taxi driver and is aware that seizures must be declared to the DVLA. On questioning, the patient denies having a seizure, he says he swerved to avoid another car. He asks to leave the department without assessment. He has capacity.

Rank the following responses in order from most appropriate to least appropriate.

a.   Warn the patient that you are obliged to tell the DVLA that he might have had a seizure.
b.   Try to encourage the patient to inform the DVLA if he thinks there is any chance he has had a seizure.
c.   Discuss the case with your consultant and call the MDU for legal advice.
d.   Discharge the patient as he has capacity and you have no evidence that he has had a seizure.
e.   Explain that everything he tells you is confidential and it is important he stays for at least a CT scan to rule out any serious pathology.

Best answer: c
Senior and legal advice are needed as this is a complex situation
Worst answer: a
This is threatening a patient with limited information, which is appropriate
Middle answers: b, d, e
This is another difficult legal case and must be dealt with by a senior. As a foundation doctor (c) is the only reasonable answer. (b) is more appropriate than (d) as you have made some effort to consider the safety of the public. (e) is less appropriate as you are being dishonest with the patient – if you discover a

brain tumour in his temporal lobe you may well have to break confidentiality and inform the DVLA. (a) is least appropriate as you are breaking confidentiality and being dishonest (before talking to your consultant and the MDU you should not be contacting the DVLA).

7. The phone rings on the ward for a long time and no one seems to answer it. It's your first day as an F1 and you think it will be a good idea to pick it up. It's Mrs Miggin's daughter asking for an update. Mrs Miggin had her hip replacement surgery 2 days ago and is recovering well.

Choose the top three most appropriate actions from the list:

a.   Explain that her mother is doing well and there is nothing to worry about.

b.   Ask if she would like to speak to her mother's nurse who has spent a bit longer with her today.

c.   Confirm that it is indeed Mrs Miggin's daughter by asking for her mothers address, date of birth and presenting complaint.

d.   Explain that you cannot divulge patient information over the phone for confidentiality reasons.

e.   Go to ask Mrs Miggin for her permission to divulge medical information about her over the phone to her daughter.

f.   Take a phone number and offer to call the daughter back if her mother agrees to you giving her medical information out over the phone.

g.   Pretend you do not know Mrs Miggin because you have forgotten the rules regarding confidentiality.

h.   Ask her daughter instead to come in during visiting hours and you can talk to her in person, with her daughter's permission.

Eliminate as clearly wrong: a, b, g
These all break confidentiality, lie or defer the problem
Best answers: c, e, f
This is quite a common scenario and one that causes relatives great frustration if you try to explain that you cannot divulge confidential data without the patient's permission. There are many anecdotes about journalists calling hospital wards pretending to be the relatives of high profile patients. It is prudent to try to confirm the identity of the person on the end of the phone (c). Elderly patients are often eager for you to update their children (f), but this must only be done with their permission (e). Do not pass the phone to the nurse without the patient's consent (b), and do not lie (g). Some relatives live long distances from the hospital and visiting (h) is often impractical and not necessary in this case.

8. You are seeing a patient in A&E who is 17 years old with intellectual disability. She has been brought in with abdominal pain. You initially see her with her carer who then leaves to get a cup of tea. Whilst they are gone you continue to ask questions and when asked about sexual activity she says that she has sex with her

carer but asks you to promise not to tell anyone. What should you do? Pick the 3 most appropriate answers:

a. Promise her you wont tell anyone
b. Confront the carer and ask if this is true
c. Do a pregnancy test
d. Explain that you will need to tell someone
e. Perform a forensic examination
f. Ask the patient if she wants to talk further about this
g. Do a capacity assessment on the patient
h. Get your senior involved

Answer: D, C, H

Eliminate clearly wrong: A, B, E. Promising not to tell is a lie, confrontation is unlikely to add anything especially in ED and you are not qualified for a forensic exam.

Reasoning
This is a difficult situation. You will need to tell someone (d) and you cannot lie to the patient and say you wont. She is in with abdominal pain and needs a pregnancy test (c). Your senior needs to be involved as there are large safeguarding issues (h).

F and G although not wrong are not within the three best purely as they are less urgent or do not cut as quickly to the result as D, C and H.

8. On your walk through the car park you find a patient list with confidential information about your current inpatients. It has your SHOs handwriting over it.

Rank the following responses in order from most appropriate to least appropriate.

a. Take the list home with you and burn it.
b. Return to the hospital with the list and dispose of it using a confidential waste bin, inform your team about the incident in the morning handover meeting.
c. Return to the hospital with the list and dispose of it using a confidential waste bin, ask your SHO whether they had lost their list when you see them tomorrow.
d. Return to the hospital with the list and dispose of it using a confidential waste bin and complete an incident form.
e. Take the list home and bring it back tomorrow to show the SHO.

Best answer: c
This is the quickest and most direct way to address both the lost list and the person likely to have lost it

Worst answer: e
Although not a terrible option this does not destroy the list and so is worst
Middle answer: b, d, a
The most appropriate answer is (c), you may be mistaken about who had los the list and seeking information is never a bad idea. The least appropriate answer is (e) as you are not destroying the list. Answer (c) is less appropriate than (b) as you should not be returning to the hospital to complete paperwork during your time off. Answer (a) is less appropriate still because you risk losing the list on your journey home.

9. One of the medical registrars who emails you a spreadsheet containing sensitive patient information. The spreadsheet is not password protected and has been sent to you personal email account so that you can work on it from home.

Rank the following responses in order from most appropriate to least appropriate.

a.　　Assign a password to the document, delete the original email and send it back to the registrar. Text the registrar the password.
b.　　Delete the email and explain that you will work on the database from a hospital computer.
c.　　Delete the email and ask the registrar to resend the document to your NHS email address.
d.　　Delete the email and purchase an encrypted memory stick to transfer the data securely.
e.　　Anonymise the data by replacing the patient names with their hospital numbers

Best answer: b
This ensures the data is safe any never leaves approved computers
Worst answer: c
Although better than your personal account this does nothing to address the patient identifiable information being off site and not secure.
Middle answers: d, a, e
Ideally patient data should not leave the secure hospital computers and therefore most appropriate answer is (b). While (c) is the least appropriate answer as you have made no attempt to secure the data you have merely sent it to another email address. If patient data is to be transferred it must be done so via an encrypted device (d). It is difficult to chose between (b) and (e). Under new confidentiality guidelines hospital numbers are no longer considered anonymous by the GMC and therefore (a) is more appropriate as it adds an element of security to the document.

4.4   Capacity

Capacity to consent is a medical judgement and is assessed formally by the ability to:
Understand
Comprehend risks and benefits
Retain information
Make a decision based on all the information
This is covered by the Mental Capacity Act 2005, and all adults are assumed to have capacity until proven otherwise. If a patient is deemed to lack capacity then the doctor should always act in the best interest of that patient without discrimination and try to involve the patient wherever possible.

10. You are working in the medical admissions unit when a patient with a history of dementia comes in with severe dehydration kidney failure. She is refusing all treatment.

Rank the following responses in order from most appropriate to least appropriate.

a.   Discuss patient's wishes with her next of kin to see if this was something she had felt strongly about before and if they had views on treatment
b.   If you deem her incapable of making decisions treat under common law
c.   Review the notes to see if there is an advanced directive in place or anticipatory care plan
d.   Assess the patient's capacity yourself to judge whether she can refuse treatment
e.   Let her refuse treatment and send her home

Best answer: d
Capacity is a decision specific concept so you would need to asses her for this particular choice
Worst answer: e
Assuming she has capacity is wrong as this could be delirium and not her dementia and very different to her expressed wishes before. You need to perform a thorough assessment before making any decisions.
Middle answers: c, a, b
This question deals with communication in difficult circumstances and capacity assessment. Although the patient has a history of dementia you don't know how advanced this is and she may still have capacity to make decisions about her treatment thus the first thing you need is to make a brief assessment of her capacity (d) by whether she is able to understand the information you give her, retain it and communicate it back to you. If you deem her to not have capacity and you feel this is an emergency you can treat her under common law without detaining her (b). However if she does not have capacity you should look and see if there is an anticipatory care plan in place (c) for this kind of situation to say that she would not wish to be treated, but this would not be appropriate if she still has capacity. (a) would be helpful if the patient does not have capacity

TOPICS

or an advanced directive in place, however family members can often change their minds when a patient becomes acutely unwell. (e) may be appropriate once you have gone through other options and feel that this is acting in the patient's best interests but you absolutely cannot do this until there is a clear plan from patient or family. In reality if there is any doubt you are much safer to treat the patient from a legal perspective.

11. You are the FY1 on the renal ward and one of your patient's blood results from the morning has shown a marked hyperkalaemia at 7.1mmol/L. This is the 4th time this has occurred for this patient in the last 3 days. You check with the lab and the sample was not haemolysed. You initiate the hyperkalaemia treatment as per your hospitals guidelines. You recheck the patient's blood a little while later and he is still hyperkalaemic at 6.5mmol/L and has now started to show ECG changes. You speak to the registrar who advises you on further management, including blood tests. You attend to the patient and explain the situation however, the patient clearly states that he no longer wants treatment and wishes to be left alone. The patient has capacity.

Rank the following responses in order from most appropriate to least appropriate.

a.   Call the patient's next of kin and ask them to persuade the patient
b.   Ignore the patient's wishes and initiate the management plan
c.   Accept the patient's wishes and pursue no further treatment
d.   Talk to the patient to explain all the risks of not receiving the treatment, as well as the reasoning behind the treatment
e.   Document in the notes that the patient has refused

Best answer: d
It would be most appropriate to explain the situation to the patient in more detail, as he may not have fully understood the gravity of the situation. This would then give the patient a chance to make a fully informed decision.
Worst answer: b
Ignoring the patient's wishes is least appropriate, and can be classified as assault of the patient if an invasive action is performed.
Middle answers: a, e, c
By asking the next of kin to discuss the matter with the patient (A), you may be able to improve the patient's understanding of their diagnosis and the necessary treatment. It is always good medical practice to document all your conversations with patients and their relatives in the notes (E) and is more appropriate than just accepting the patient's wishes (C) without first seeking to improve the patients understanding, as you cannot be certain the patient is fully aware of the details of the situation therefore this must be clarified. Moreover, (E) would also help to inform your colleagues of the situation.

4.5   Consent

Consent is 'permission or agreement for an action to occur'. This covers a wide range of procedures, and a junior doctor must only consent patients for what they are able to do. When in doubt a senior colleague should consent the patient.

When the patient is a child, there are other considerations to take into account. The Family Law Reform Act 1969 states that those over the age of 16 has the same ability to consent to treatment as anyone over the age of 18. This however does extend to refusal of treatment, and would require involvement of seniors and the hospital's legal team.

Gillick competence refers to a child under the age of 16 who is deemed able to consent if they have demonstrated 'a sufficient understanding and intelligence to be capable of making up their mind on the matter requiring decision' without the need of parental consent.

With young people who lack capacity, consent should be obtained from a parent. This matter is complicated if there is disagreement, which if cannot be resolved informally, will require legal advice.

12. As the F1 on your general surgery job the consultant asks you to consent a patient for an incision and drainage of an abscess under local anaesthetic that is happening tomorrow. You have seen a couple of these procedures before and vaguely understand the complications include recurrence, bleeding and scarring.

Rank the following responses in order from most appropriate to least appropriate.

a.   Explain to the consultant that you are not comfortable taking consent for the procedure, offer to find the registrar to take consent and ask to join the consultant in theatre so that you can learn how to take consent in future.
b.   Attempt to take consent.
c.   Print off a patient information leaflet and go through it with the patient before obtaining consent.
d.   Agree to take consent, talk through the procedure with the patient, then ask the registrar to check the form and sign it.
e.   Agree to take consent but hand the task over to the on-call SHO at the end of your shift.

Best answer: a
This avoids taking a consent you are not qualified to take and gives you the opportunity to learn to be able to do so in future and help your team
Worst answer: b
This would be invalid as you are not competent to actually do the procedure
Middle answers: d, e, c

You are not competent to take consent in this scenario and should not attempt to do so. Therefore (a) is the most appropriate answer and (b) is the least appropriate. (d) is the next most appropriate after (a) because the registrar is likely to retake consent for you. (e) is less appropriate than (d) because the on-call SHO may not be competent to take consent, or might not have time to. (c) is slightly more appropriate than (b), but reading a patient leaflet does not make you competent to take consent!

4.6 | Raising Concerns

All juniors should familiarise themselves with their local trusts policy about raising concerns, and this is covered in the GMCs Good Medical Practice 2013. In the SJT common scenarios include
-       Health, behaviour or professional performance of a colleague
-       Any aspect of the environment where treatment is provided
-       Being asked to do something that conflicts with a doctors duty to put patients' interests first and/or to act to protect them
Concerns may be raised with;
-       Senior colleagues
-       Clinical/educational supervisors
-       Foundation programme dean
-       Head of departments
-       Medical defence organisation
-       CQC
-       GMC
There should be an open policy for raising concerns.

A handy mnemonic for dealing with concerns is "SPIES"
-       Seek info – you need to understand the problem
-       Patient safety – always your first priority
-       Initiative – what can be done immediately?
-       Escalate – inform the relevant parties
-       Support – ensure individuals and teams have access to support

13. The ward matron has come to you as she has noticed multiple pieces of equipment missing from the storeroom. Later that same week you walk into the storeroom to find your colleague putting various IV access equipment into their bag.

Rank the following responses in order from most appropriate to least appropriate.

a.   Leave the store room without mentioning anything and continue on with your day
b.   Report your colleague to the ward matron
c.   Confront your colleague and question them about what you have noticed
d.   Inform your colleague's clinical supervisor of what you have seen

e.   Ask advice from your registrar

Best answer: c
Upholding honesty and integrity is one of the 4 main principles outlined in the GMCs 'Good Medical Practice'. The most appropriate option is to seek more information about the situation by talking to the colleague in question privately (C), there may be an explanation as to why he is doing what you have seen.
Worst answer: a
Not telling anyone of what you have seen and ignoring the situation (A) is least appropriate as it shows a complete lack of integrity with regards to a situation that you have been asked to be aware of.
Middle answers:
If you are unsure what to do it is appropriate to speak to a senior staff member for advice (E) as they may have experience on the matter. Considering the ward matron has flagged the issue to you earlier in the week, they should be informed (B) of what you have witnessed so that they are able to follow up on it. This is more beneficial than going to your colleague's clinical supervisor (D), as the ward matron is the most relevant point of contact (she is the person in control of the ward). The clinical supervisor should be informed at some point, so that they are able to follow up with the colleague, but it is not your immediate priority.

14. At a mess party your registrar offers you some cocaine. You are surprised because at work he is extremely professional and you have never had concerns about his care for patients.

Rank the following responses in order from most appropriate to least appropriate.

a.   Politely decline and go home.
b.   Politely decline but in the morning talk to the registrar and try to ascertain whether his cocaine use is purely recreational or whether he are suffering from dependency or mental illness.
c.   Politely decline and discuss the matter with your consultant.
d.   Report the registrar to the police and the GMC.
e.   Report the registrar to the GMC.

Best answer: b
Dealing with the issue head on at a neutral time is the best way to explore the situation and decide if anything needs to be done
Worst answer: d
Represents a knee jerk reaction without much knowledge behind it in what could be a difficult situation and could cause a lot of trouble for both you and the registrar
Middle answers: c, a, e
In this question it is important to think about what your actions will actually achieve. The most appropriate answer is (b). Cocaine use may be a manifestation of mental illness and the registrar may need professional help. It is always wise to seek more information in SJT scenarios. The least appropriate answer is

(d) because this may be career ending for your registrar and you currently have no reason to believe his actions are adversely affecting patient care or that he is involved in serious criminal activity. (e) is slightly more appropriate as with this response he will only have to deal with a GMC investigation as opposed to a GMC investigation and a police investigation. In doubt your consultant will be a good port of call (c) but it would be prudent to talk to the registrar first. Your consultant is likely to have more experience than you in dealing with such matters. (a) is a completely neutral response.

15. You are an F2 in the Emergency Department. The police bring in a 19 year old man, under arrest, who they suspect is in possession of class A drugs. He admits to you that he swallowed a large amount of cocaine, loosely wrapped in cling film, to avoid the police finding it. He asks you not to tell the police. He wants to be discharged and declines to have the cocaine removed. He understands that he might die and has mental capacity to make this decision.

Rank the following responses in order from most appropriate to least appropriate.

a.   Discharge the patient documenting the conversation clearly in the medical notes. Do not provide a copy of the discharge summary (which would incriminate the patient).
b.   Discuss the situation with the consultant and contact the MDU for legal advice.
c.   Explain that you will have to divulge this information to the police as it is in his best interests to be brought back should he start to feel unwell.
d.   Hand the police a copy of the discharge summary in a sealed envelop signed 'medical notes, in confidence'. Explain that this is a confidential document, which needs to be read by the medical officer in the detention centre, but not by the police, and cannot be used as evidence. Tell the patient you have done this and document the conversation clearly.
e.   Discuss the case with the registrar.

Best answer: b
In a complex situation getting both senior and legal advice is appropriate
Worst answer: c
In a competent patient this is a breach of confidentiality
Middle answers: e, d, a
This is a complex situation and must be dealt with by a consultant. The only acceptable answers are (b), and (e) the registrar is likely to talk to the consultant and contact the MDU). The MDU is likely to give advice along the lines of response (d), which strikes a balance between your duty of confidentiality and your duty to share important medical information with other carers. Answer (a) does not break confidentiality, but is potentially dangerous because you have not warned the healthcare professionals at the police station that the patient is at high risk of cocaine toxicity. Answer (c) is the least appropriate answer. The patient has capacity and is capable of deciding what is in their best interests.

In this response you break confidentiality and have no guarantee of getting the medical details across to the custody team at the police station.

4.7   Gifts

With regards to accepting gifts, the GMC states that 'You must be honest and open in any financial arrangements with patients'. You must assess the situation in a professional manner, and patients should be made aware they are not obliged to reward you for your services, and that it does not impact on the quality of care provided

16. You are the FY1 on the Geriatric ward and you have been caring for Mr Jones, an 89 year old gentleman for the last 2 months. He is finally ready to go back home when you are approached by his son. His son offers you a personal cheque for the amount of £50 (written with your name on it) as thanks for looking after his father.

Rank the following responses in order from most appropriate to least appropriate.

a.   Accept the cheque. The patient's son is very insistent and you agree that you have been integral to the patient's return to health
b.   Politely decline the cheque informing the relative that it would be inappropriate for you to accept it and politely direct him to the ward matron instead so that he can leave positive feedback for the ward
c.   Politely decline the cheque but explain to the son that there is a ward charity that does accept donations. You explain that if he would like more information he should speak to the ward matron but he should in no way feel obliged to donate
d.   Explain to the son that it would be better for him to buy chocolates for the ward as everyone contributed to his father's care
e.   Accept the cheque as to not offend the son but quickly dispose of it. Inform the ward staff of the relatives gratefulness

Best answer: b
The most appropriate option would be to politely decline the cheque and allow him to leave positive feedback (B). This would maintain the professional relationship between yourself and the relative.
Worst answer: a
The GMC states; "You must not encourage patients to give, lend or bequeath money or gifts that will directly or indirectly benefit you". Therefore, accepting the cheque for your own gain is the least appropriate option.
Middle answers: c, d, e
By making the son aware of the ward charity, but not putting pressure on him to donate (C), you are allowing the son to show his gratitude if he would still like, without persuading him, which would be against GMC principles of 'Good Medical Practice'. This would be more appropriate than suggesting the son use the money to buy chocolates for the ward (D), as this could be construed as a coercion that would ultimately benefit you (in violation of the GMC rules).

TOPICS

Accepting the cheque even with the intention of discarding it (E) would be inappropriate as it is dishonest and could lead to a breakdown in the relationship between yourself and the son, by falsely reassuring him it is acceptable to take monetary gifts.

4.8 | Work/life balance

'Good doctors make the care of their patients their first concern', and you have a duty to ensure there is appropriate cover and handover for patients. This allows commitments outside of work, and working excessive hours will impact on patient care. However, it is important to note, that if cover has not been arranged, it is in the patients' be interests you remain until you are suitably relieved from your duties, despite the risk of mishap due to hours worked rather than having no cover.

17. You are the F1 on a care of the elderly ward. It is Friday night, and you are enjoying some well-earned rest in the pub after a long 12-day stretch. Suddenly you remember you have forgotten to put blood forms out for the weekend for Mr X, a 94-year-old gentleman who had a severe AKI today. Do you:

a.   Ring the hospital switchboard, ask to bleep the ward cover F1 and then ask them to put blood forms out for the weekend.
b.   Repeat the blood tests on Monday
c.   Message your friend who you know is covering a different ward over the weekend and ask them to put the forms out tomorrow.
d.   Go back into work tonight to out the forms out yourself.
e.   Call the ward, ask the nurses to remind the F1 covering the ward to put out bloods tomorrow.

Best Answer: A
This deals with the problem quickly with a direct handover which is the safest.
Worst Answer: B
A severe AKI per the question is likely to need review over the weekend a this could compromise the patients care.
Middle answers: C, E, D

In this scenario you have not completed your jobs properly, and patient safety is at risk. Notice the question specifies a severe AKI and the patient could be very unwell if left until Monday, therefore option B is the least acceptable.
Option A is the best course of action, although the F1 will probably be busy you have officially handed over the job, and it is now their responsibility to make sure the blood forms are put out as they are covering that ward, and hand over that the results need chasing over the weekend. Option C will likely result in the patient having the tests, but these will not necessarily be acted upon as your friend is not covering that ward.
Option E is not acceptable, it is not the nurses job to hand over tasks you forgot to the ward cover doctor. Option D is not a good idea, particularly if you have been in the pub!

18. You are on your last shift of a busy set of nights. You have not slept well during the day as your neighbours are in the middle of a noisy loft conversion. By 0400 you become very tired, the nurses have made you doubt some of your management plans and you notice you are starting to make prescribing errors because you are sleep deprived.

Rank the following responses in order from most appropriate to least appropriate.

a.   Take a break, have a strong coffee and leave less urgent tasks for the day team.

b.   Take the batteries out of your bleep and have a 30 minute nap.

c.   Inform the registrar. Handover the list of patients you have seen and potentially made mistakes with. Divert your bleep to her and go to sleep in an on-call room until you are safe to make the journey home. The time you have had off will need to be registered as sick leave.

d.   Continue with the shift and ask the day team to do detailed reviews of the patients you saw overnight

e.   Inform the registrar. Hand her your bleep so that you can sleep for a couple of hours.

Best answer: c

If you really are unsafe you need to remove yourself from the clinical environment

Worst answer: d

Review could be over 5 hours away and if you are making errors harm may come to your patients in the interim

Middle answers: e, a, b

It is important to recognize when you are unfit to work. The most appropriate answer is (c). Your registrar will need to review the patients you have potentially put in harm's way. In the scenario the consultant might have to be called in from home to help cover the wards in your absence. (e) is less appropriate because you are unlikely to be fit to practice after 2 hours more sleep. The least appropriate answer is D as you are continuing to put patients at risk. (b) is slightly more appropriate as you are attempting to address your tiredness, but removing the batteries from the bleep will also put patients at risk. (a) is slightly more appropriate than (b) because you are attempting to address your fatigue without losing contact with the team. Answers (a, b, d) are all highly inappropriate.

19. It is 17:30 and you have just finished your shift, which was supposed to finish at 17:00. You are just about to leave the hospital, and suddenly get a call from the nurse on your ward who says that she needs a patient looking at immediately as they have suddenly deteriorated. She tells you that the on-call doctor has not yet turned up to the hospital. You are in a bit of a rush as you are scheduled to meet your family for dinner, who have travelled up on the train to visit you.

Rank the following responses in order from most appropriate to least appropriate.

a.   Tell the nurse that your shift is over and it is no longer your responsibility
b.   Ask the nurse to call the registrar on-call
c.   Return to the ward, assess and stabilise the patient and leave a plan in the notes for the on-call doctor for when he arrives
d.   Inform the site coordinator of that the on-call doctor has not yet turned up
e.   Return to the ward, assess and stabilise the patient and wait for the on-call doctor to arrive

Best answer: e
Although not ideal this is your responsibility until it can be safely handed over
Worst answer: a
This is bad for patient care and potentially dangerous
Middle answers: c, b, d
As a doctor you have a duty of care to your patients, and although an emergency may happen outside of your rota'd hours you are required to attend to this and manage the patient appropriately. In this instance, there is currently no doctor on-call and your priority is patient safety; therefore, you must attend to the patient (b) and (e) and (c). Once you have stabilised the patient it is better for you to wait for the on-call doctor to give him a verbal handover (e), than it is to just leave him a plan in the notes (c), as he may not see these straight away. These are both better than just getting the nurse to inform the registrar on-call (b), as in the time it takes her to do this and for the registrar to attend, the patient could have deteriorated further. Also, the registrar may be busy with other patients. Informing the site coordinator (d) is helpful for them so that they can chase the doctor, but in no way will help the patient in their current predicament. Telling the nurse that it is no longer your responsibility is both incorrect and places patient safety at risk (a).

20. You are working on a busy orthopaedic ward and often leave late due to the workload. One of your fellow FY1s is interested in orthopaedic surgery and often goes to theatre during the day leaving you to deal with the heavy workload alone.

Rank the following responses in order from most appropriate to least appropriate.

a.   Speak to the consultant to see if you can devise a fair rota rotating all the FY1s into theatre or clinic when there are enough staff on
b.   Agree a plan with the FY1 that he can go to theatre but if the workload becomes unmanageable you will bleep him
c.   Speak to your clinical supervisor about concerns regarding the workload
d.   Let him go to theatre during the day but handover all the outstanding jobs to him when he gets back so that you can leave on time

e.   Speak to the FY1, explain your concerns and that the workload should be split evenly giving you equal opportunity to go to theatre but that the ward takes priority if it is busy.

Best answer: e
Unfortunately as an F1 your job can be largely administrative, sometimes at the detriment of your clinical experience. It is not fair in this scenario to be left to do the work alone. Equally regardless of future aspirations, opportunities to learn should be shared equally. This option addresses these points well

Worst answer: d
This avoids the issue by deferring the work until after theatre. Staying after work should never be planned for and adding extra handovers could introduce errors. It also deprives you of valuable learning opportunities

Middle answers: a, c, b
Trying to get teaching opportunities is important during your training but ultimately your ward work and patients take priority. Even if you are not interested in orthopaedic surgery, theatre and clinics are still important learning experiences and it is not fair for you to take on the workload yourself and so therefore the best option is (e) to try and negotiate a fair rota amongst yourselves so that you all manage the workload and get equal teaching opportunities. If it does not get resolved speaking to the FY1 directly you should try and crate a fair rota with the consultant (a). If you are struggling with the workload your clinic supervisor can help (c) but if the only reason you are struggling is because you are short staffed because another FY1 is shirking ward responsibilities then you should try and resolve this first. (b) and (d) are both inappropriate as you are missing out on valuable teaching experience and neither of you should be leaving late if at all possible.

4.9 | Complaints

Complaints are often a result of a series of smaller events, contributing to overall patient dissatisfaction. The GMC states that you must "respond promptly, fully and honestly to complaints and apologise when appropriate". Be aware of local complaint processes and how to direct patients to the relevant teams i.e. Patient Advice and Liaison service.

21. You are cornered in the corridor by an angry relative who is shouting that his mother is not being looked after properly and is demanding to know what is wrong with her.

Choose the three most appropriate actions to take in this situation

a.   Meet with your patient first to ensure that she is happy that you share information about her admission with her son

b.   Tell the patient to stop shouting on the ward as he is making the doctors look bad

c.   Explain to the relative that you cannot meet with him because of confidentiality reasons and that he will just have to ask his mother

d.   Politely ask the patient not to shout as he is disturbing other patients and say that you will meet with him in a quiet room away from other patients and relatives.

e.   Explain to the relative that if he has a complaint he can put it in writing

f.   Ask the patient politely to keep his voice down and then explain to him what is wrong with his mother and what she is being treated for

g.   Call security to have him removed from the ward

h.   Take another member of staff with you to meet with the family member to ensure there is a witness if the family member remains angry, becomes violent or makes a complaint about you

Best answers: a, d, h
Eliminate as clearly wrong: b, e, g
This question deals with your professionalism under pressure. Although you may be intimidated you need to remain professional, need to protect your patient's confidentiality and also ensure he is not distressing other patients. As such you need to remain polite and courteous, asking him to lower his voice and agreeing to meet with him to discuss his concerns away from where you can be overheard (d), however before you do this you need to be sure that your patient, who should always remain your priority, is happy for you to share her information with her family (a). Lastly to protect yourself, you need to take a chaperone so that if a complaint is made you have a witness and it is not your word against theirs (h). Refusing to speak to him and having him removed from the ward is only going to exacerbate the situation (b, c, g) and sharing confidential information in front of other patients and families is wholly unprofessional (f) even if it does help diffuse the situation.

4.10 | Treating friends and family

The GMC advises that you must avoid treating yourself or anyone you have a personal relationship with. However, if you find yourself in a situation where it is necessary to manage someone close to you, you must treat them as you would any other patient.

"Good Medical Practice" states that you must maintain a professional boundary between you and your patient. This will include your social media presence, and so be sure to read the GMC's "Doctors' use of Social Media", prior to the exam.

22. While using an online dating app. You get along well with one of your matches and become very fond of them, but it soon dawns upon you that they were a patient of yours, four months ago during a busy surgical rotation. They ask you to go on a date with them.

Rank the following responses in order from most appropriate to least appropriate.

a.   Politely explain that you cannot pursue your romance further as this would be deemed unprofessional by the GMC.

b.   Contact your indemnity company for legal advice.

c.   Go out on the date, you are no longer obliged to maintain professional boundaries as your doctor-patient relationship ended four months ago.
d.   Cease all communication with your former patient and block them from the app.
e.   Ask your former patient what they think about the situation.

Best Answer: b
This represents the safest option in a murky situation
Worst answer: c
This ignores the potential issues without addressing them at all
Middle answers: a, d, e

The GMC guidance on personal relationships with former patients is not clear or universal. Such relationships may be inappropriate depending on the length of time since the professional relationship ended, the nature of the previous professional relationship, whether the patient was particularly vulnerable at the time of the professional relationship, whether they are still vulnerable and whether you will be caring for other members of the patient's family. It is best to contact the MDU for legal advice in these situations (b). Without further information about your professional relationship the least appropriate answer is (c). Answers (a) and (d) both end your personal relationship with the former patient but (d) is unnecessarily rude. You are unlikely to gain impartial advice by asking what your former patient thinks (e).

23. You are an F2 working in the Emergency Department. One of your colleagues, another Emergency Department F2 who is on annual leave, has booked in as a patient. There is currently a three-hour waiting time. Before seeing the triage nurse he catches you in the department and asks if he could skip the queue. He says he only needs a replacement salbutamol inhaler and his consultation will be a very quick one.

Rank the following responses in order from most appropriate to least appropriate.

a.   Ask one of the nurses to grab your colleague a salbutamol inhaler from the drug cupboard and let him go on his way.
b.   Explain to your colleague that he will have to wait three hours as seeing him immediately would not be fair to the other patients.
c.   Stop what you are doing, a detailed history from your colleague and perform an examination, prescribing the inhaler if necessary, and document everything clearly in your colleague's medical records.
d.   Make a brief ABC assessment. If your colleague is having an acute exacerbation of asthma he made need escalating, if not he will have to join the waiting list.
e.   Explain that there is a three hour wait, and offer to call his mobile phone when it is nearly his turn to be seen so that he can leave the department for a while.

TOPICS

Best answer: d
While we can presume he has no significant airway compromise he may still be quite unwell with an infective exacerbation of asthma. Do not be reassured by his assessment of himself.

Worst answer: a
Drugs should never be handed out in the Emergency Department without a history, examination and adequate documentation including prescriptions.

Middle answers: e, b, c
E is more appropriate than B as you are he might find the gesture of telephoning him kind and that will improve your working relationship. C is less appropriate as you are potentially putting other patients at risk by stopping what you are doing, and skipping the queue is unfair to other patients in the waiting room. (d) and (a) will both jeopardise your working relationship with your consultant but (d) is more likely to put an end to his behaviour.

Tips before moving onto the supplied 70 question mock paper

Ranking questions – pick the best and worst answers first. Then if time complete the remaining three as best you can. However do not dwell on these.

Multiple choice – make sure that you only select 3 answers, and that these are the best three in your opinion.

In the supplied mock we suggest you complete using the available marking sheet under strict timed conditions - stick to 2 minutes per question.

Remember that although there are 70 questions, only 60 are 'live' so account for this when marking.

TOPICS

5 MOCK SJT

MOCK SJT

1. **You are the FY1 in the Respiratory Team. You go to find the consultant in his office as he has not yet turned up for ward round. As you approach his office you hear him shouting at your CT1 colleague, who subsequently runs out looking very distressed.**

Rank the following responses in order from most appropriate to least appropriate (1= Most appropriate; 5= Least appropriate).

a.   Don't think anything more of it and inform the consultant he is needed on ward round

b.   Confront the consultant straightaway regarding his behaviour towards your colleague

c.   Inform your Clinical Supervisor of the event

d.   Continue to inform the consultant of the ward round and once the ward round has finished have a talk with your CT1 colleague regarding the situation

e.   Immediately go and check on your colleague

2. **You are the SHO on-call in General Surgery on the weekend and a 15-year-old girl has come in with severe RIF pain. An ultrasound scan of the abdomen shows inflammation surrounding the appendix and a diagnosis of appendicitis is given. Having performed appendicectomies in the past, you are asked to consent the patient for surgery, but have found that the parents are refusing the procedure.**

Rank the following responses in order from most appropriate to least appropriate (1= Most appropriate; 5= Least appropriate).

a.   Assess the patient for Gillick Competence, and proceed to consent the patient if found to be Gillick Competent

b.   Perform the procedure as it is in the best interests of the patient, despite the parents refusal

c.   Ask your registrar for advice

d.   Discuss the procedure with the parents further, to try to persuade them

e.   Inform the consultant that the patient is not consenting.

3. **You are the surgical FY1 in a DGH on call. You have just clerked in an unwell patient with an acute abdomen requiring immediate surgery. Your registrar has seen the patient and asked you to call the consultant in to take the patient to theatre. The on-call consultant says he has had 3 glasses of wine but he is going to drive into the hospital and will be 30 minutes. What is the most appropriate action to take?**

Rank the following responses in order from most appropriate to least appropriate (1= Most appropriate; 5= Least appropriate).

MOCK SJT

a.   Call another consultant in to do the surgery
b.   Postpone the surgery until the morning
c.   Tell the theatre that the surgery will start in 30 minutes
d.   Go and pick the Consultant up so he does not have to drive
e.   Immediately write an email to the GMC saying the consultant has been drinking on call

4.   You are working in Accident and Emergency and have just seen a patient who requires admission. They have presented with confusion and bloods show a severe AKI with uraemia and hyper-kalaemia. She has a GCS 10/15. Her past medical history shows that she is known to the urology team with bladder cancer which was close to obstructing the ureters when she was last seen 4 months ago. You refer her to the urology team who refuse to come to see the patient as she has presented with confusion and an AKI – a medical problem. You speak to the medical team who say that it is a urology cause for the problem and so a urology problem. What is your next step?

Rank the following responses in order from most appropriate to least appropriate (1= Most appropriate; 5= Least appropriate).

a.   Speak to your senior about immediate interventions
b.   Tell the family that the patient is not able to come into hospital
c.   Call urology and insist that they accept the patient
d.   Call the renal consultant to ask for the patient to be dialysed
e.   Write to the CEO of hospital about patient flow

5.   You are the FY1 on ward cover and a nurse calls you saying a patient wishes to self-discharge. You have not met this patient before but after having a quick read through the notes you understand that he is here for an infective exacerbation of COPD with possible underlying lung ca. He has no other PMH and no mental health issues documented. You go and talk to the patient and he is sitting patiently on the end of his bed stating that he wishes to go home as he is not allowed out for cigarettes. He is orientated to time, place and person. What is the next most appropriate step?

Rank the following responses in order from most appropriate to least appropriate (1= Most appropriate; 5= Least appropriate).

a.   Order an immediate CT head looking for brain metastasis
b.   Physically restrain the patient to the bed
c.   Allow the patient to sign self-discharge form in the presence of yourself and a nurse

d.   Discuss the risks of the patient going home against medical advice and assess his capacity

e.   Call your SHO and ask them to come and see the patient

6.   A nurse gives you the phone stating that the relatives are on the phone for one of your patients asking to speak to the doctor. You answer the phone and there is a female voice shouting at you. She says that she is the daughter of a patient whom you know well on the ward. She is upset and angry that no one has called her to tell her what is happening with her mother. From previous conversations with the patient you are aware that she has not spoken to her daughter in many years. What is the most appropriate course of action?

Rank the following responses in order from most appropriate to least appropriate (1= Most appropriate; 5= Least appropriate).

a.   Put the phone down

b.   Tell the daughter on the phone what is happening with the patient immediately

c.   Go and ask the patient what information she would like you to tell her daughter, if any

d.   Give the patient the phone

e.   Tell the daughter on the phone that she will need to call back tomorrow

7.   You are the surgical FY1 and have been asked to help with the take as it has been a busy afternoon. You clerk a patient who has an abscess on their right thigh which is starting to become uncomfortable. It is red and has an area of fluctuance of around 3cm. The patient has previously had an abscess on the other thigh and is asking you to "cut it and let the pus out" just like they did last time. He is getting more and more agitated the longer he is waiting on the trolley and starts to shout. You have read about I&D in text books but never seen or done one yourself. What should you do next?

Rank the following responses in order from most appropriate to least appropriate (1= Most appropriate; 5= Least appropriate).

a.   Chemically sedate the patient

b.   Use a scalpel to Incise and drain his thigh

c.   Use a needle to drain the abscess

d.   Call your SHO to come and review the patient and drain the abscess

e.   Start the patient on antibiotics

8.   An elderly lady who has been your patient on the elderly care ward for the last few weeks. She was suffering from a chest

infection and died over the weekend. You came to know her and her husband well and had many conversions with them over the course of her stay. The following Monday the patients husband comes back to the ward with a card for you and a large box of chocolates. He insists on you taking the gift and has given another box of chocolates to the nurses. What should you do?

Rank the following responses in order from most appropriate to least appropriate (1= Most appropriate; 5= Least appropriate).

a.   Accept the chocolates and share them with the team
b.   Take the chocolates home and eat them with your housemates
c.   Apologise and refuse the chocolates
d.   Declare the chocolate gift to the GMC
e.   Accept the chocolates as a gesture and thrown them in the bin

9.   You are the FY1 on elderly care medicine at a tertiary hospital. An 84 year old gentleman previously independent and living alone has recently had a CT abdomen and pelvis for abdominal discomfort and bloating, which showed possible lesion on the pancreas. Your consultant asks you to contact the Hepatobiliary team for review of the patient. The registrar says that they are too busy to see old people. What should you do next?

Rank the following responses in order from most appropriate to least appropriate (1= Most appropriate; 5= Least appropriate).

a.   Ask the surgical registrar on call for review
b.   Wait until tomorrow and try again, hopefully someone else will be on call
c.   Tell the consultant you were unable to get a hold of them
d.   Ask your registrar if they would make the call
e.   Ask your consultant to call the HPB consultant

10.   You are the FY1 on a busy surgical firm and your fellow FY1 who was supposed to be on post take with you has called in sick for the last 2 days. The take has been busy and you have stayed late over 2 hours each night. You check your Facebook when you get home and see that your fellow FY1 has been tagged in some photos in a long weekend in Croatia. He is back at work the following day, what do you do?

Rank the following responses in order from most appropriate to least appropriate (1= Most appropriate; 5= Least appropriate).

a.   Not say anything
b.   Take your college aside and talk to him

c.   Inform the GMC of his deception
d.   Email his educational supervisor to tell him what has happened
e.   Take the next two days off and leave him to do the work

11.   You are the FY1 on general medicine. A gentleman has been admitted with haemoptysis and weight loss, he had a high-resolution CT this morning and the report is of probable small cell lung cancer with local lymph node enlargement. As you pass him he asks about his scan results. What should you do?

Rank the following responses in order from most appropriate to least appropriate (1= Most appropriate; 5= Least appropriate).

a.   Tell the patient you do not know the result of the scan
b.   Explain to the patient that it will be discussed on the ward round by the consultant
c.   Tell him he may have cancer but you cannot say much more without your consultant
d.   Ask him to have a family member present before the results are discussed
e.   Ignore the patient and continue walking past

12.   You are the FY2 in a GP surgery and have just started doing your own clinics. You see on the list of patients for the day that there is a patient who you know from outside work. This makes you uncomfortable. What should you do?

Rank the following responses in order from most appropriate to least appropriate (1= Most appropriate; 5= Least appropriate).

a.   Say you feel sick and go home
b.   Ask your supervisor to see the patient instead
c.   Ask reception to cancel the patient's appointment
d.   See the patient
e.   Ask your supervisor to chaperone you

13.   You are the FY1 on elderly care and one of your patients has been placed on the end of life pathway. They have been started on a syringe driver with morphine and diazepam. She appears comfortable and in no distress. Her daughter is present and from America, she asks how long it will take for her mother to die. She says that in America they just increase the morphine until she passes and why can you not do that. What should you do?

Rank the following responses in order from most appropriate to least appropriate (1= Most appropriate; 5= Least appropriate).

a.   Increase the morphine PRNs on the drug chart

b.   Stop the syringe driver
c.   Explain to the daughter that she is comfortable and it will be increased if needed
d.   Increase the diazepam in the syringe driver
e.   Offer to discuss the medications with the consultant

14.   You are on a surgical firm who are on take. There is an 8 year old whom you are concerned has acute appendicitis. The school nurse and his teacher have brought him to hospital and they have been unable to contact his parents. He is unwell and not responding to fluids well. Your senior is currently consenting the child and the teachers. What is it important to consider?

Rank the following responses in order from most appropriate to least appropriate (1= Most appropriate; 5= Least appropriate).

a.   The child can be consented under guardianship act
b.   The parents need to be informed
c.   The teachers can consent for him in his best interests
d.   You need to wait until the parents have consented to do the surgery
e.   The surgery can take place in the patients best interest

15.   You are the medical FY1 and the daughter of one of your patients comes to talk to you. You know her mother, an 89 year old who is currently being treated for pneumonia. The daughter is holding a DNACPR and says that someone has put this on her mother and it should not have been. She says wants her mother treated and does not want you to try and kill her. She wants the DNACPR revoked. What should you do?

Rank the following responses in order from most appropriate to least appropriate (1= Most appropriate; 5= Least appropriate).

a.   Revoke the DNACPR
b.   Tell the daughter it is a medical decision and cannot be changed
c.   Discuss with the daughter what the DNACPR means and explain that it will not stop treatment
d.   Discuss with the patient and the daughter the patient wishes
e.   Call your consultant and ask them to come to the ward

16.   You have been called by a nurse on the ward asking you to come and do a cannula so a patient can have their evening dose of antibiotics, which is due now. You are currently seeing a patient with an acute abdomen who you feel may need surgery. What should you do next?

Rank the following responses in order from most appropriate to least appropriate (1= Most appropriate; 5= Least appropriate).

a.   Call your senior to do the cannula
b.   Call your senior to come and review the patient you are seeing
c.   Leave immediately to go and do the cannula
d.   Ignore the call about the cannula and continue what you are doing
e.   Tell the nurse on the phone you will be there once you have finished what you are doing

17.   You are just starting a new firm on surgery and you have been added to a WhatsApp group by your fellow FY1, also on surgery. They tell you that the surgical registrars put the patient information of the patients they clerk each day on the WhatsApp so that you can add them to the list, that way no patient is forgotten about. What should you do?

Rank the following responses in order from most appropriate to least appropriate (1= Most appropriate; 5= Least appropriate).

a.   Check the patients have been added to the list from today
b.   Report this to your educational supervisor
c.   Remove yourself from the group
d.   Ask for only patient numbers to be added to the group
e.   Report each member of the group to the GMC

18.   You are the surgical F1 on call, seeing patients in the surgical assessment unit on take with the surgical registrar. A patient you had seen earlier with the registrar can be discharged with antibiotics and analgesia. You ring the registrar, who is in theatre, who asks you to discharge the patient with an FP10 prescription.

Rank the following responses in order from most appropriate to least appropriate (1= Most appropriate; 5= Least appropriate).

a.   Ask the registrar to suggest analgesia and antibiotic doses and complete the FP10 yourself
b.   Take the FP10 form to theatre for the SpR to complete
c.   Complete a FP10 for antibiotics and analgesia as per local guidelines and the BNF
d.   Try and find the surgical SHO to complete the prescription
e.   Refuse to complete the FP10 as F1s are not authorised to do so

19.   You are the F1 on nights, on your first weekend of medical ward cover. You have been bleeped to the respiratory ward to see an unwell patient. An experienced nurse says she has seen patients like this receive a theophylline infusion, and suggests you do the same. You have not prescribed a theophylline infusion before and are unfamiliar with how to do so. You bleep the medical

registrar who does not respond. The patient continues to deteriorate.

Rank the following responses in order from most appropriate to least appropriate (1= Most appropriate; 5= Least appropriate).

a.   Bleep the medical registrar again and wait for their advice
b.   Look up theophylline infusions on the trust intranet.
c.   Dial 2222 and put out a peri-arrest call
d.   Bleep the F2 on call for advice
e.   With the nurse's help write up the infusion and review the patient again in 15 mins

20.   You are the surgical F1 and have been asked by the consultant on call to assist with a nephrectomy as the registrar and SHO are busy. The patient has been anesthetized and the consultant is about to begin when you realise the consent form stated left kidney, but the consultant is about to begin on the right-hand side. You try to raise this with the consultant who tells you, you are incorrect.

Rank the following responses in order from most appropriate to least appropriate (1= Most appropriate; 5= Least appropriate).

a.   Take off your glove and desterilise the consultant.
b.   Leave it there, the consultant is much more experienced, and is probably correct and you are mistaken.
c.   Raise your concern with the anaesthetist.
d.   Ask the ODP to find the consent form and show it to the consultant.
e.   Wait until the consultant reaches the kidney & then restate your concerns, hopefully he will then notice he has the wrong side.

21.   You are the F1 on a general medical ward, and have been involved in the care of a patient with longstanding back pain, who has been on the ward for some time and is now medically fit for discharge. The consultant has explained on numerous occasions that her scans have not revealed any acute pathology, and management will involve physiotherapy and analgesia. You are seeing the patient on an F1 ward round when she demands your GMC number, stating she wishes to make a complaint about you specifically for "not taking her back pain seriously", and "trying to throw her out without a cure'.

With regards to her ongoing care, do you:

Rank the following responses in order from most appropriate to least appropriate (1= Most appropriate; 5= Least appropriate).

a.   Refuse to see the patient again
b.   Refuse to see the patient and ask your SHO to see them instead.
c.   See the patient again, only with a nurse chaperone
d.   Tell your colleagues not to see the patient either, she is MFFD
and blocking a bed, hopefully this will encourage her to leave.
e.   Continue seeing the patient alone, as you do not want to inconvenience you colleagues.

22.   You are the F1 on weekend ward cover and have been asked to take blood samples from a patient for gentamicin levels. He is an IVDU and difficult to bleed; the phlebotomists have failed to collect a sample this morning and have asked you to do it. You have met the gentleman before and have also been unable to get a blood sample from him in earlier in the week. Do you:

Rank the following responses in order from most appropriate to least appropriate (1= Most appropriate; 5= Least appropriate).

a.   Call the ward cover SHO and ask them to take the sample
b.   Take an arterial sample without trying to take a venous sample first
c.   Call the 3rd Anaesthetist on call and ask them to take the sample
d.   Attempt to take a venous sample
e.   Do nothing, the sample is only for antibiotic levels and can wait until Monday.

23.   You are an F2 on medical nights, and it is around 3am. A patient with severe learning difficulties you saw together with the medical registrar is deteriorating rapidly, and the management plan is now for best supportive care. The registrar asks you to document everything, as she has to rush off to see another unwell patient in A&E. As you are filling in the DNACPR form you notice there is a box that states "has this form been discussed with the family"? Do you:

Rank the following responses in order from most appropriate to least appropriate (1= Most appropriate; 5= Least appropriate).

a.   Complete the form, do not discuss with anyone.
b.   Telephone the family and ask for their views and only complete the form if they agree.
c.   Complete the form, then immediately call the family to inform them the decision has been made
d.   Complete the form, and at handover ask the ward team to telephone the family first thing in the morning
e.   Do not complete the form, and at handover ask the ward team to telephone the family first thing in the morning and complete the form if the family agrees.

24. Whilst standing at a Nurses Bay in the middle of a busy ward a middle grade doctor tells you and a few of the nurses a joke he heard on TV last night, from a comedian with a known preference for suggestive jokes. There are a few laughs and then you go to review some of the ward patients. Your first patient is in a bay close to the Nurses station and when you greet her she asks for the name of the staff member who told the joke as she found it offensive and wants to make a complaint.

Rank the following responses in order from most appropriate to least appropriate (1= Most appropriate; 5= Least appropriate).

a.   Explain to the patient that it was a joke from National TV and that the Doctor was only repeating it with no intention to offend.
b.   Apologise to the patient and give her the name of your colleague
c.   Explore the patient's feelings and offer to bring in a Senior Nurse to have a chat about making a complaint
d.   Tell the patient you weren't there when the joke was told and possibly it was a delivery man or another relative who told a joke.
e.   Excuse yourself politely, fetch the middle-grade doctor and ask them to apologise and have a chat with the patient to avoid a complaint.

25. Whilst working as an FY1 on a surgical ward you notice than one of your FY1 colleagues is not washing his hands between examinations of patients. He is handling notes, computer terminals and his own mobile phone in this time.

Rank the following responses in order from most appropriate to least appropriate (1= Most appropriate; 5= Least appropriate).

a.   Point the fact out to your colleague on the next Consultant ward round to show your team that you are taking Infection Control seriously
b.   Ask the Senior Nurse to have a chat with him about proper infection control as you don't want to damage your working relationship
c.   Suggest to your consultant that the ward undertake an audit of Infection Control techniques during surgical ward rounds
d.   Speak to your colleague directly about what you have observed
e.   Make an obvious show of washing your hands between patients and hope that your colleague takes the hint.

26. An FY1 colleague of yours who is very keen on medical education has made a WhatsApp group with some medical students. As you are keen to gain some teaching experience she adds you to this group to help organise sessions. As part of the group you realise that your colleague is sharing identifiable details of patients over the group to allow the students to find them in the hospital and examine them.

Rank the following responses in order from most appropriate to least appropriate (1= Most appropriate; 5= Least appropriate).

a.   Exit the group immediately as you do not want to be implicated in any trouble that may arise.
b.   Raise your concerns with your colleague's clinical supervisor but request that your name is kept out of it
c.   Accept your colleague's assurances that WhatsApp messages are secure and encrypted and therefore patient confidentiality is not at risk.
d.   Seek advice from your defence union
e.   Canvass opinion from FY1 colleagues about whether this is an appropriate use of patient details.

27.   During the first few months as an FY1 on an acute medical rotation you have become aware that some of your peers are adapting less well than others to the role and responsibilities of being a doctor. One FY1 colleague confides in you that they have been crying on their drive into work every morning as they think about how stressful the job is.

Rank the following responses in order from most appropriate to least appropriate (1= Most appropriate; 5= Least appropriate).

a.   Talk through their feelings and reassure them of their capability and dedication as an FY1.
b.   Offer to cover of their upcoming long days so they can take annual leave and have a break.
c.   Recommend they speak to their Educational Supervisor about these issues.
d.   Tell the other junior doctors on the rotation not to burden your colleague with too many jobs as she is having trouble coping.
e.   Speak to the Acute Medicine consultant in confidence about the issues your colleague has raised.

28.   As part of your FY2 rotations you are placed at an inner-city GP surgery with a large patient population. After a short settling in period you are asked by your GP supervisor to perform daily home visits to housebound patients. You don't feel 100% confident performing these assessments alone particularly in complex medical patients and let your supervisor know of your concerns. Your supervisor's response is that supervising doctors cannot be spared as they have their own visits to perform, and as long as you debrief on the visits afterwards you will be fine.

Rank the following responses in order from most appropriate to least appropriate (1= Most appropriate; 5= Least appropriate).

a.   Stand your ground and refuse to perform any further home visits without supervision

b.   Request that your supervisor only sends you out to see cases that sound straightforward on phone triage

c.   Accept that your supervisor knows best and continue as previously although you still harbour concerns and worry that you are not giving some patient's optimum care

d.   Discuss the matter with your educational supervisor

e.   Raise the issue with another senior partner at the practice who is not your clinical supervisor

29.   At your work Christmas party your FY2 colleague is visibly drunk despite being on-call tomorrow from 8am. You also know that they drive at least 30mins to work each morning and are concerned that they won't be fit to make the drive safely tomorrow morning.

Rank the following responses in order from most appropriate to least appropriate (1= Most appropriate; 5= Least appropriate).

a.   Stay out of the matter, it's not your place to comment on someone's behaviour outside of work

b.   Speak to one of the Consultants at the party about your concerns

c.   Keep a close eye on them and keep a tally of how much they drink over the course of the night

d.   Take your colleague aside and remind them of their shift tomorrow and suggest they might need to take a Taxi.

e.   Ask the bar staff to ensure that no further drinks are served for the doctor in question thus saving any embarrassment.

30.   You arrive for work on a busy acute surgical emergency unit and realise that you forgot to put the blood forms out correctly yesterday and none of the patients have had their bloods done ahead of the consultant ward round.

Rank the following responses in order from most appropriate to least appropriate (1= Most appropriate; 5= Least appropriate).

a.   Ask a couple of the nurses to help and start bleeding the patient's yourself before the rest of team arrive

b.   when the consultant arrives tell them that there has been a problem with the computer system and it means the bloods were not done

c.   Bleep the phlebotomists, explain your error and ask them if they could return to the ward and do the bloods

d.   Explain to your consultant that you forgot to do the bloods and blame how hard you have been working saying the duties expected of you are unreasonable

e.   Apologise to your consultant when they arrive, offer to make sure the bloods are all done later and call the consultant with the results

31.   You are one of two FY1s on a medical team. While you get on well with your colleague personally you can see that they are struggling with the workload. In order to ensure the smooth running of the ward you are taking on more and more of the work. One day your clinical supervisor takes you aside and tells you she has noticed that your teaching attendance is well below 50% and asks you why this is.

Rank the following responses in order from most appropriate to least appropriate (1= Most appropriate; 5= Least appropriate).

a.   Apologise to your consultant, say it is your fault and that you will endeavour to make all future sessions and do e-learning on topics you have missed

b.   Be honest with your consultant and tell them you have been covering for your colleague as you think they are struggling

c.   Say nothing to give your colleague away but resolve to only do your share of the work from now on and attend teaching every week

d.   Ask your consultant to get in a locum as the workload is too much for 2 people

e.   Take the blame for missing sessions and continue to help cover for your colleague as they are your friend and the sessions you have been to were boring anyway.

32.   On joining your new rotation, you realised that your consultant and senior registrar do not see eye to eye. Their working relationship has continued to deteriorate and now, once the consultant has left following ward rounds, the registrar ridicules the plans made by the consultant and recommends you follow his suggestions instead.

Rank the following responses in order from most appropriate to least appropriate (1= Most appropriate; 5= Least appropriate).

a.   Ask that the Registrar raises his concerns about the plans directly with the consultant as you are uncomfortable ignoring direct instructions

b.   Ask a consultant on a nearby ward which plans would be most appropriate to follow

c.   Follow the registrar's suggestions but document clearly in the notes that it was his decision to change the original plan

d.   Call the consultant and tell them that the registrar feels their plans are inappropriate

e.   Ignore your registrar's comments and follow the original consultant plans

33.   As the FY2 on General Surgery you regularly consent

patients prior to elective laparoscopic cholecystectomies and your consultant allows you to perform most of the procedure under their supervision. While consenting a patient before a morning list the patient tells you that he only wants the consultant to perform his surgery, as he doesn't trust trainee surgeons.

Rank the following responses in order from most appropriate to least appropriate (1= Most appropriate; 5= Least appropriate).

a.   Inform the patient that they cannot choose who they want to be treated by and if they don't like that they can cancel their operation.

b.   Ask the consultant to come and discuss the operation with the patient

c.   Agree to the patient's wishes and take no part beyond assisting in the surgery

d.   Humour the patient and but ask to perform the operation as normal once the patient is asleep

e.   Explore why the patient does not trust trainee surgeons and explain it is the only way to train the consultants of the future

34.   **You are reviewing the post-take patients with your consultant on the morning round. You receive a bleep from your ward asking you to return there urgently to insert a cannula, as a patient is due IV antibiotics and their last cannula tissued overnight. When you ask if anyone there could do it instead the nurse abruptly tells you that they are too busy and she will document that the doctor was informed but refused to come.**

Rank the following responses in order from most appropriate to least appropriate (1= Most appropriate; 5= Least appropriate).

a.   Your professional relationship with the nurse

b.   The timely administration of the ward patient's antibiotics

c.   The opinion of your consultant on the post-take ward round

d.   Ensuring your side of the story is documented in the notes

e.   Finding out why the cannula was not replaced by the overnight staff

35.   **You become concerned that one of your colleagues is becoming too attached to one of the patients on the ward. This patient has a terminal illness with a poor prognosis and your colleague goes to speak with them every day after work and often leaves looking visibly upset.**

Rank the following responses in order from most appropriate to least appropriate (1= Most appropriate; 5= Least appropriate).

a.   Advise your colleague to seek counselling from Occupational Health or their GP

b.   Tell your colleague they need to harden up or they will suffer a break-down
c.   Email their clinical supervisor and inform them of your concerns
d.   Take your colleague aside and find out more about the visits to the patient and voice your own concerns
e.   Take no action as what a colleague does outside of working hours is not your concern.

36.   Your friend at work tells you that his leave request has been rejected as there is not enough cover. However, he intends to call in sick regardless as he is a groomsman at his best friend's wedding. Sure enough a week later he calls in sick. Your consultant comes to you and asks where your colleague is as the ward is very short-staffed.

Rank the following responses in order from most appropriate to least appropriate (1= Most appropriate; 5= Least appropriate).

a.   Tell your consultant the truth, that he has called in sick in order to attend a wedding
b.   Tell your consultant you don't know anything about it apart from that he has called in sick
c.   Suggest to your consultant that they call your colleague themselves if they want more information
d.   Tell your consultant that he had been looking very peaky yesterday and is most likely off sick
e.   Offer to work a long day to get all the jobs done as best you can.

37.   You have just received the results of a CT scan on a patient, Mr Munroe, just before the end of your shift. You know he was keen to hear the result and go to inform him of them before you leave for the day. When you arrive, you find that Mr Munroe is asleep in the presence of his daughter-in-law. You explain why you have come and Mr Munroe's daughter-in-law suggests you tell her the results and she can tell him when he wakes up.

Rank the following responses in order from most appropriate to least appropriate (1= Most appropriate; 5= Least appropriate).

a.   Wake Mr Munroe up and tell him the scan report before you go
b.   Tell his daughter-in-law the scan report and ask her to relay the details when Mr Munroe awakens
c.   Print off a copy of the scan report and seal it in an envelope for Mr Munroe to read when he awakens.
d.   Hand over to the doctor on ward cover that evening to visit Mr Munroe later and tell him the scan report
e.   Apologise to his daughter-in-law and explain that for confidentiality reasons you will visit Mr Munroe early tomorrow to relay the results in person.

38.   You are called to see a delirious patient overnight. You see a plan written by your day-time FY2 on the consultant ward round in case of such a scenario which recommends a dose of sedation which you know to be several times higher than the usual starting dose. No written justification is given for the higher dose.

Rank the following responses in order from most appropriate to least appropriate (1= Most appropriate; 5= Least appropriate).

a.   Give the dose as suggested by the ward round note.

b.   Bleep the on-call registrar for their advice

c.   Change the plan and give the regular starting dose of the sedative as recommended by the BNF

d.   Ask the nursing staff what dose is normally given to delirious patients on the ward

e.   Call your FY2 on their mobile to ask why the higher dose has been recommended

39.   You are a Foundation Trainee working in A&E. Your consultant asks you to contact the Neurosurgical Registrar on-call to discuss the results of an MRI Spine with him. The imaging revealed no changes since the last scan 6 months ago. While on the phone, the registrar begins belittling and shouting at you for what he believes to be an inappropriate referral.

Rank the following responses in order from most appropriate to least appropriate (1= Most appropriate; 5= Least appropriate).

a.   Replace the phone handset immediately as bullying should not be tolerated in the workplace

b.   Shout back at him telling him that his behaviour is unacceptable

c.   Wait for the phone conversation to end, do not mention anything to him or any of your colleagues about the incident

d.   Explain to him on the phone that you do not think his tone is appropriate, bear with the conversation then raise the issue with your Clinical Supervisor at an appropriate time

e.   Wait until the conversation is over then immediately contact your clinical supervisor as it has caused you significant distress

40.   You are a Foundation Year 1 trainee working on an infectious diseases ward. Your registrar asks you to perform a lumbar puncture on one of the patients because she is busy in clinic and the Core Medical Trainee (CMT) did not answer her phone five minutes ago. You have never done a lumbar puncture being performed but you have observed two.

Rank the following responses in order from most appropriate to least appropriate (1= Most appropriate; 5= Least appropriate).

a.   Explain that you will only do the lumbar puncture if adequate supervision is available as you have never done one before and try to get hold of your CMT to supervise you
b.   Explain that you will do the lumbar puncture and contact the registrar if you come across any difficulties
c.   Refuse to do the lumbar puncture as you lack the experience to do so
d.   Offer to take responsibility of ensuring the lumbar puncture is done but find someone else to do it instead of you and observe them performing the procedure
e.   Refuse to do the lumbar puncture but offer to continue trying to get hold of the CMT to do it while you do your ward jobs

41.   You are a Foundation Year 2 doctor and have cared for Dorothy, an 86 year old patient, who has been an inpatient on your ward for over 117 days. She is due to be discharged tomorrow morning to a residential home. After the ward round the day prior to her discharge, she calls you over personally and informed you she has a small gift of appreciation. She starts counting out £200 cash and informs you she asked her son to bring it from her savings.

Rank the following responses in order from most appropriate to least appropriate (1= Most appropriate; 5= Least appropriate).

a.   Kindly thank her for the warm gesture but refuse to accept the money
b.   Accept the money and place it in the ward fund for future staff outings
c.   Accept the money as a personal token of appreciation of your work over the past four months
d.   Refuse to accept the money but inform her if she would like to leave feedback for the care she has received, direct her to the PALS team
e.   Refuse to accept the money but inform her she can donate the £200 to the ward if she so chooses

42.   You notice that your FY1 colleague has been taking pictures of clinical signs from patients on your ward and sharing them on a public social media educational group he has formed for the final year students. He tells you the group is growing and he has been recruiting medical students from other schools. In addition, he said he has been using it as a platform to educate the public and does not deny anyone access to the group. He tells you he has been getting verbal consent from the patients.

Rank the following responses in order from most appropriate to least appropriate (1= Most appropriate; 5= Least appropriate).

a.   Speak to him in person explaining that his use of social media might be against GMC guidance

b.   Inform him that if he wants to continue it he should seek advice from his Clinical supervisor as he may

c.   Suggest he may need ethical approval and written consent for such an undertaking

d.   Suggest he takes down all pictures and does not upload or take any more until advice is sought from a senior

e.   Explain that his teaching scheme is a good idea and that you would be willing to help expand it by taking more pictures for the teaching group

43.   You are a Foundation Year 1 doctor on a busy general surgical ward. Officially you start at 7:30am daily however the lists are expected to be printed and stapled ready for the consultants at that time. As such you have been arriving half an hour early daily to deal with the lists. The other four FY1 colleagues have not taken this role upon themselves and as such you are always the one in early to do the lists and you all leave at the same time. You are now two months into rotation.

Rank the following responses in order from most appropriate to least appropriate (1= Most appropriate; 5= Least appropriate).

a.   Continue to print the list without mentioning your grievances

b.   Refuse to come in early to print the lists and let the entire team of juniors deal with the consequences

c.   Mention your concern to your FY1 colleagues

d.   Discuss your concern with your clinical supervisor

e.   Devise a plan for each FY1 to print the list a different day of the week

44.   You are a Foundation Year 2 doctor on a GP rotation. One of the patients whom you regularly see with mental health problems, Jenny, has requested to be your friend on a social media platform. Alongside the request is a personal message in which Jenny explains how much your care has changed her life for which she is extremely grateful.

Rank the following responses in order from most appropriate to least appropriate (1= Most appropriate; 5= Least appropriate).

a.   Reject the request refuting Jenny's message and telling her it would not be appropriate for you to see her as a patient again

b.   Accept the request and respond to Jenny with a message thanking her for her kind words but emphasizing that you are just doing your job

c.   Accept the request but delete her as a friend the following day

d.   Reject the request explaining to Jenny you do not think it appropriate or professional to be friends on social media

e.   Ignore the request

45.   You are a Foundation Year 2 doctor working in A&E. A pa-

tient, Eleanor, comes in intoxicated and having taken recreational drugs. She becomes aggressive and threatens to physically abuse staff.

Rank the following responses in order from most appropriate to least appropriate (1= Most appropriate; 5= Least appropriate).

a.   Try to calm Eleanor down using de-escalation techniques
b.   Call security
c.   Refer Eleanor to substance misuse services
d.   Re-hydrate Eleanor to help her sober using intravenous fluids
e.   Medically sedate her using appropriate therapy

46.   You are a Foundation Year 1 trainee working on a busy surgical ward with 70 patients on the list. You are doing your morning ward round with the team. The consultant asks your F1 colleague, Greg, to prescribe a medicine for one of the patients which he does so immediately. Later that afternoon when going through the ward round jobs, you check his prescription and realize that he prescribed the wrong drug; one that the patient was allergic too, but had not yet been administered.

Rank the following responses in order from most appropriate to least appropriate (1= Most appropriate; 5= Least appropriate).

a.   Complete a serious incident form
b.   Inform the nurse caring for the patient to not administer the drug
c.   Cross the drug off the drug chart
d.   Prescribe the correct intended drug
e.   Speak to Greg in private and inform him of the mistake

47.   You are have just got home from a busy shift and make a cup of tea and log on to Facebook. A colleague from work has posted a photo of themselves scrubbed up in an operating theatre, you are not friends with them on Facebook but a friend of yours has liked it. The patient on the table is not visible however behind your colleague is the list of patients with visible patient details and operation due for the rest of the list. Choose the three most appropriate actions to take in this situation

a.   Report the photo to Facebook
b.   Message your colleague and tell him what you have spotted
c.   Write a comment underneath the photo
d.   Report the photo to the colleague's educational supervisor
e.   Report you colleague to the GMC
f.   Ignore it and continue your Facebook browse

g.   Ask your friend who is friends with the person in photo for their number so you can call them and tell them of the breach in confidentiality

h.   Remind the colleague at work that they need to tell their educational supervisor in case the photo appears in a complaint or the media.

48.   Your grandmother sadly passes away and the funeral is subsequently arranged for next week. You quickly realize you are on call Monday to Thursday on long days. You ask medical staffing and your consultant if you can take it as bereavement leave but they say they have no cover so you cannot. You are upset but able to carry on your jobs but obviously want to go, how should you address the issue? Choose the three most appropriate actions to take in this situation

a.   Complain to medical staffing again

b.   Threaten to involve the BMA

c.   Call in sick on the day

d.   Try and find a colleague yourself to swap with

e.   Offer to pay for a locum yourself

f.   Ask to compromise and just have the middle of the day off and return for the evening on call after the funeral

g.   Escalate to hospital management

h.   Attend your on call as planned

49.   You are an F2 doing A and E in a busy department over winter. You find you are often needed to ask questions and your seniors are busy but usually of great help when you do ask. However, one consultant often berates you for asking "stupid questions" and "not having a plan, expecting me to solve your problems" before giving any advice. You find this difficult and upsetting as you are working hard and trying your best in often difficult circumstances. How best should you address this? Choose the three most appropriate actions to take in this situation

a.   Where possible avoid that consultant and ask others for help

b.   Continue as before hoping you may learn what he wants and stop being so annoying

c.   In a quieter moment ask him for some feedback and how he would suggest you improve?

d.   Report him for bullying

e.   Ask your clinical supervisor for help dealing with the matter

f.   Take it upon yourself to make more decisions yourself without asking for help

g.   Ask around your colleagues to see if he treats them the same

h.   Try to swap off shifts where he is working

50.   You have just started your second rotation as an F1, and are working with another F1 you have not met previously. Over the first two weeks, she is consistently late for work, leaving you to prepare the list alone in the mornings. You also notice her frequently leaving the ward rounds for 5 mins at a time. When you confront her about this she confides in you she is pregnant, but begs you not to tell anyone else as she does not want her parents to know. Choose the three most appropriate actions to take in this situation

a.   Tell her to speak to her GP
b.   Keep her secret – do not tell anyone
c.   Speak directly to her clinical supervisor.
d.   Explain to your consultant why she is always late.
e.   Encourage her to speak to her educational supervisor
f.   Ask the F2 on your firm to come in early to help with the list
g.   Offer to cover some of her duties over the next few weeks
h.   Speak to your educational supervisor for advice.

51.   It is the first few weeks of your first placement as an F1, and you find you are frequently staying late to finish off jobs left over from the ward round.

Choose the three most appropriate actions to take in this situation

a.   Ask some fellow F1s for advice about job prioritization
b.   Skip F1 teaching to help complete jobs on time on the busy ward
c.   Ask the SHO to help with a greater proportion of the jobs, they are always leaving at 5pm
d.   Knuckle down and keep working hard, all F1 jobs are like this
e.   Start coming in earlier to complete jobs from the day before
f.   Speak to your educational supervisor about managing your workload
g.   Raise your concerns with your consultant on the ward round
h.   Speak to your clinical supervisor about managing your workload

52.   You are the F1 on a busy gastroenterology ward, and the consultant points out that one of your patients requires an ascetic tap. You have not seen or performed this procedure before.

Choose the three most appropriate actions to take in this situation

a.   Ask your registrar to perform the procedure
b.   Ask the SHO if they are able to perform the procedure
c.   Ask your registrar if they are able to supervise you performing the procedure
d.   Ask your registrar if you can observe them performing the procedure
e.   Perform the procedure with a nurse chaperone

MOCK SJT

f. Research the procedure on the internet
g. Collect all the equipment required for the procedure
h. Consent the patient for the procedure

53. It is the last day of your F1 year and you are working as the general surgical F1. You have been given the unenviable task of chasing up all the outstanding histology results of discharged patients before the new F1 intake begin work tomorrow. Towards the end of the day you find a routine appendicetomy sample from a few months ago is reported as a showing evidence of a possible malignancy. You have not met the patient before.

Choose the three most appropriate actions to take in this situation

a. Telephone the patient directly to inform them of the result
b. Contact the patient's GP to inform them of the result
c. Email the consultant who was looking after the patient of the result
d. Hand over to the new surgical F1s to follow up on the result
e. Speak to the local gastrointestinal cancer specialist nurses and arrange for them to follow up on the result
f. Draft a letter to the patient to inform them to make an appointment with their GP to discuss the result
g. Hand over to the surgical registrar
h. Ask the secretaries to arrange an urgent follow up appointment with the consultant.

54. It is a Friday night, and you are on a ward cover shift. You are the F1 passing through a ward when a nurse asks if you can urgently rewrite a drug chart for a patient. They have recently moved wards and their drug chart has been misplaced. When you enquire why the drug chart needs rewriting urgently the nurse informs you that the patient is due to newly start chemotherapy tomorrow, and this was prescribed on that chart.

Choose the three most appropriate actions to take in this situation

a. Call the oncologist on call overnight and ask for the correct chemotherapy doses
b. Review the medical notes and use them to prescribe the chemotherapy
c. Rewrite a chart with analgesia and the patient's regular medications on for use overnight.
d. Hand over for the day team to contact the patient's consultant in the morning to organise the chemotherapy
e. Attempt to prescribe the chemotherapy from the medical notes yourself
f. Ask the medical registrar on call to prescribe appropriate chemotherapy
g. Ask the patient if they can remember the drug name, and prescribe from the BNF.

h.   Help the nursing staff search for the missing original chart.

55.   You are a Foundation Year 1 trainee working on a gastro-enterology ward. One of the young female patients is extremely grateful for the care she has received and attributes thanks to you as the ward doctor. She compliments your work outfit today and asks if you are single. She then proceeds to ask you out for a meal after she is discharged this afternoon.

Choose the three most appropriate actions to take in this situation

a.   Accept their offer of a meal as a sign of gratitude and meet them after work

b.   Reprimand them and tell them that their behaviour is completely inappropriate and unacceptable

c.   Explain to them you do not think this is appropriate given that you have been caring for them in a position of trust and responsibility

d.   Kindly thank the patient but refuse to accept their offer without further explanation

e.   Suggest going for a drink might be more appropriate and invite some of your friends to make it less personal

f.   State that you are busy but that your FY1 peer might be free this evening to accompany them

g.   Inform the patient you would not feel comfortable going out with them for a meal because of the negative perception this may have on doctors to the public

h.   Inform the patient you will ask you consultant and get back to them

56.   You are a Foundation Year 2 doctor on a general surgical ward. One of the registrars and the consultant are scrubbed in theatre and get the theatre staff to bleep you and ask you to consent the next patient for an open subtotal colectomy. You have assisted in doing the operation once before.

Choose the three most appropriate actions to take in this situation

a.   Contact your other registrar who is finishing the ward round to consent the patient once the ward round is finished

b.   Consent the patient to the best of your ability and knowledge based on the information you remember from assisting in the procedure

c.   Ask the theatre staff to apologize to the consultant and registrar that you do not feel competent enough to consent the patient

d.   Acknowledge the theatre staff request but do not consent the patient, wait till they finish in theatre and then tell them you did not have time to consent the patient

e.   Offer to go and scrub in theatre to free up the registrar to consent the patient for the next operation

f.   Find out as much information regarding the operation from reputable

MOCK SJT

resources such as peer-reviewed journal articles and established surgical text-books prior to consenting the patient yourself

g.   Ask your fellow FY2 colleague to come and consent the patient with you so that between you the majority of the information can be addressed

h.   Refuse to consent the patient but have the consent form ready with the patient details on it so that when finished in theatre, the registrar can quickly consent the patient

57.   You are a Foundation Year 2 doctor working in A&E. Half way into your shift, your ex-partner, presents as a patient and is demanding that you come and medically assess them in the hope they can reduce their waiting time and get back to work as soon as possible. One of the A&E nurses has come to tell you this information while you are seeing another patient.

Choose the three most appropriate actions to take in this situation

a.   Go and see them immediately and tell him this is inappropriate

b.   Ask the nurse to tell them you are currently seeing another patient

c.   Call security as you feel uncomfortable with them in the department

d.   Ask the nurse to explain to them that patients are seen in order of time of arrival into the department and on the basis of clinical need

e.   Make sure another clinician sees them as your clinical judgment may be impaired by your knowledge and previous experiences with them

f.   See them when they is the next to be seen in time of arrival into the department

g.   Ignore the information that the nurse gave you and make sure you are on your break when he is next to be seen to avoid assessing him

h.   Complete a serious incident form

58.   You are a Foundation Year 2 doctor working in A&E. The nurses have been trying to contact the gynaecology team for an hour to come and see a young female patient who is clearly in a lot of pain having been referred in by her GP. She has been unable to do so and as a consequence the patient has not had any analgesia prescribed. She has now been in A&E for one and a half hours. The nurse approaches you to prescribe some analgesia for the patient until the gynaecology team come to assess her. You are good friends with the gynaecology SHO due to see her.

Choose the three most appropriate actions to take in this situation

a.   Refuse to prescribe anything as the patient is not your clinical responsibility

b.   Refuse to prescribe anything as the patient may be nil by mouth if requiring emergency surgery

c.   Prescribe appropriate analgesia

d.   Offer to rapidly assess her to identify the extent of the problem and whether she needs to be seen immediately in light of possible gynaecological emergencies

e.   Offer to bleep the gynae SHO yourself

f.   Escalate the fact the patient has not been seen and has been waiting in pain to your A&E consultant in charge

g.   Ask the surgical team to come and see her instead

h.   Ask your A&E colleague with an interest in gynaecology to see her

59.   You are a Foundation Year 1 doctor. You are in an elevator with three nurses from your ward and family of Angela, a patient on your ward, who are visiting. The nurses, not knowing the passengers in the elevator are Angela's family, start making jokes about Angela's care needs and who she has been drooling on herself since having a stroke. You notice that Angela's family are visibly upset at what they are hearing but do not say anything at the time.

Choose the three most appropriate actions to take in this situation

a.   Ignore the incident as you were not directly involved

b.   Refute the nurses there and then in the elevator to stop the inappropriate discussion

c.   Mention Angela in conversation to the family in the hope the nurses realize they might be family and as such stop their inappropriate discussion

d.   Raise the issue with your educational supervisor

e.   Tell Angela when you get to the ward that the nurses were speaking inappropriately about her and that she may want to take up the issue with the PALS team

f.   Wait for the nurses to leave the elevator and apologize to the family, explaining what they witnessed was unprofessional and unacceptable

g.   Point the family towards the PALS team

h.   Discuss the issues with the nurses on the ward and explain to them the inappropriate nature of their discussion and the consequences that followed from the family overhearing

60.   Mrs Atkinson is an elderly lady recuperating on your ward after emergency surgery on a fractured hip. She has been making good progress and the Physiotherapists have recommended she begin walking independently with a frame. However, when you ask the nurses about her progress they tell you she hasn't been mobilising at all for two days as they can't spare a nurse to accompany her and they don't feel she is safe to walk alone.

Choose the three most appropriate actions to take in this situation

a.   Accept that the nurses know best and move on

b.   Report the nurses conduct to your consultant

c.   Arrange an MDT meeting with the physiotherapists and nursing staff to discuss Mrs Atkinson's care

MOCK SJT

d.   Stay on the ward over your lunch break so that you can accompany Mrs Atkinson while she walks on the ward

e.   Chastise the nurses and order them to allow Mrs Atkinson to walk independently

f.   Discuss the Nurses' concerns and ensure they are aware of the importance of rehabilitation after surgery to maximise functional recovery

g.   Ask Mrs Atkinson's relatives if they wouldn't mind walking with her when they visit

h.   Request that the physiotherapists perform another assessment of Mrs Atkinson's mobility.

61.   You work with another junior doctor on an elective surgical firm. You are seeing a patient when you overhear your colleague accepting a cash gift from one of the grateful patients who is about to be discharged. When you confront your colleague he breaks down and confesses that he is really struggling with personal debts and has also been borrowing money from short term, high-interest loan companies.

Choose the three most appropriate actions to take in this situation

a.   Demand he give the money back to the patient immediately

b.   Offer to lend your colleague the money he needs to clear his most imminent debts.

c.   Explain to him why he must hand over the money to the Ward Sister as a donation to the ward.

d.   Advise him to contact his Educational Supervisor to discuss the issues he is facing

e.   As it was a small amount of money tell your colleague you will overlook it this time but not to accept any more gifts

f.   Advise him to get in contact with the Citizens Advice Bureau

g.   Recommend that as long as he uses a portion of the money to buy some food or drink for the ward staff then it is OK

h.   Ask the Nursing staff to put up signs discouraging patients from giving staff members gifts

62.   The nurse in charge of your ward comes to you one morning and asks to have a chat privately. She tells you that some of the nursing staff have raised concerns with her about your attitude on the ward. She tells you that they feel you don't listen to the nurses' opinions and can often seem aloof and condescending towards them.

Choose the three most appropriate actions to take in this situation

a.   Ask for the nurses' names so you can speak to them directly about the issue

b.   Dismiss the suggestions as they are irrelevant to patient care

c.   Buy a box of biscuits for the ward staff tomorrow morning
d.   Ask the nurse for examples and talk through ways in which you could have handled the situation differently
e.   Tell the nurse in charge that being a doctor is not a popularity contest and you need to keep professional distance from your staff
f.   Ask some of your colleagues who seem to have good relationships with nursing staff for some advice and feedback on your own manner
g.   The next time you review a patient on the ward ask a staff nurse to review your plan to show you value their opinion
h.   Discuss the issue with your clinical or educational supervisor

63.   Mrs Page is due for discharge from your ward today. She has a place in a rehabilitation hospital after a long stay on the ward. Unfortunately, you get a call from the rehabilitation hospital to say that their planned discharge has fallen through and the place is no longer available. When you relay this information to Mrs Page and her family they are very upset and her son angrily accuses you of incompetence and lying to the family.

Choose the three most appropriate actions to take in this situation

a.   Assure them another bed will become available very soon
b.   Offer to call a senior doctor to come and speak to them
c.   Threaten to call security if they do not calm down
d.   Explain to the family that it is all the fault of the rehabilitation hospital
e.   Apologise to the family for the delay and attempt to calm them down
f.   Inform the family you will not tolerate abuse of any kind
g.   Offer them information on the hospitals complaints procedure
h.   Ask the nursing staff to kick them out as it is near the end of visiting hours

64.   You have been called to assist in an Emergency Caesarean Section. As you are waiting for the Spinal Anaesthetic to take effect you notice that whilst the mother looks visibly upset and anxious, across the room two of the Theatre staff are having an audible conversation about weekend plans.

Choose the three most appropriate actions to take in this situation

a.   Ask the patient if she would like the Theatre radio turned on
b.   Bring the issue up with the Theatre lead after the case to explore possible reminders/education for the staff.
c.   Make silent gestures across the room trying to Shush the theatre staff
d.   Concentrate on running through the steps of the procedure in your head to drown out the background distractions
e.   Introduce yourself to the mother and ask her how she is feeling
f.   Do nothing but confront the staff later on and lecture them on sensitivity to patient distress

g. Ask the Surgeon in charge if you can do the opening and closing of the procedure as it is a good educational opportunity

h. Quietly ask the staff to moderate their conversation as the mother looks distressed

65. Following the ward round, you notice your F1 colleague has made drug errors on at least two patients' drug charts.

Choose the three most appropriate actions to take in this situation

a. Correct the errors.

b. Apologise to the patients.

c. Take your colleague to one side and ask them about the errors.

d. Inform your consultant that your colleague has made multiple drug errors.

e. Review the drug charts of all the patients that your colleague has prescribed for.

f. Inform your colleague's educational supervisor.

g. Complete an incident form.

h. Explain to the pharmacist that your colleague is a bad prescriber and will need his work checked.

66. On a night shift, you are called to see a distressed patient. He is elderly and confused with delirium, likely secondary to a urinary tract infection. He has punched a member of the nursing staff and is wondering around the ward apparently looking for the exit. He does not have capacity to decide to leave the ward.

Choose the three most appropriate actions to take in this situation

a. Prescribe 0.5-1mg oral haloperidol.

b. Call security.

c. Talk to the patient in a calm manner and try to guide them back to bed.

d. Prescribe 0.5-1mg of intramuscular haloperidol.

e. Attend the nurse who was punched.

f. Review the patient's notes and address any other causes for his confusion (e.g. inadequate analgesia).

g. Try to stand between the patient and the nursing staff to reduce the risk to them.

h. Ask the registrar for advice.

67. 20. You overhear an F1 colleague reprimanding a nurse for not giving a patient their antibiotics on time. The patient in question overhears the exchange.

Choose the three most appropriate actions to take in this situation

a. Later on, in private, tell the F1 colleague that their actions were inappropriate.

b.   Advise the nurse to complete an incident form.

c.   Apologise to the patient and reassure them that they will get their anti-biotics on time.

d.   If you have time, ask the nurse if they need help with any of their jobs.

e.   Bring your colleague over, away from the patient and explain that the patient had heard the exchange. Recommend that they go and apologise to the patient.

f.   Bring your colleague over, away from the patient and suggest they apologise to the nurse.

g.   Inform the F1's consultant.

h.   Complete an incident form.

68.   You are the FY1 in Cardiology, and one of your patients is due to be discharged today. He was admitted due to a syncopal episode, which was secondary to a cardiac arrhythmia. This is his 2nd admission in the last 6 weeks for this. During his time in your care you have found out that he has continued to drive, despite you previously telling him that it would be unsafe to do so in his current situation.

Choose the three most appropriate actions to take in this situation

a.   Don't discuss with the patient any further

b.   Write a reflection in your ePortfolio

c.   Inform the DVLA

d.   Discuss with the patient's next of kin, to see if they are able to better explain the risks of driving to the patient

e.   Take the patient's keys from him

f.   Call the police

g.   Explain to the patient again the reasons for them not being able to drive

h.   Write a letter to the GP asking him to review the patient and to explain to them

69.   An elderly lady is admitted following a fall sustaining a fractured neck of femur. She is listed for theatre later that day but the nurses phone you to say that she is refusing to go for an operation. They say she doesn't seem to be confused but does appear very anxious.

Choose the three most appropriate actions to take in this situation

a.   Sign an adults with incapacity form (consent form 4), and tell the nurses she has no choice now she has to go

b.   Ask the patient if you can phone her family so that they can come up to the hospital and support her through this stressful time

c.   Tell the nurses you are too busy to come and see her and say the registrar will have to deal with it when they consent the patient anyway

d.   Review the patient and if you deem her to have capacity immediately refer her to a nursing home as you know she will never walk again without the operation and there are pressures on beds

e.   Phone theatre to cancel her theatre slot so that someone else can take her place

f.   Refer her to psychiatry to help with her anxiety before the operation

g.   Make your consultant aware that the patient is anxious and may not consent to theatre

h.   Put some time aside to talk her through the procedure, exploring her concerns, trying to reassure her, and making her aware of the risks if she does not have the operation.

70.   You are working as an F1 in the emergency department when you see Edna a very frail 94 year old lady with palliative lung cancer. She has presented today with a worsening productive cough. As you review her notes you see she has presented once a month for the last few months spending at least a week in hospital on intravenous antibiotics each time. Unfortunately no one has actually discussed end of life care and ceilings of care so after discussing with your consultant you sit down and have a long and ultimately very productive discussion. During this Edna and her family tell you they realise she is coming close to the end and they decide with your help that she is not for CPR and only for a trial of oral antibiotics and your consultant co-signs the form to put the treatment escalation plan into effect. Unfortunately as it is so late she cannot go home to the nursing home so she stays the night under the medical team. The next day you find an email from one of the acute medical consultants telling you that it is not your place in ED to palliate patients who can recover let alone as an F1 which obviously upsets you.

Choose the three most appropriate actions to take in this situation

a.   Reply to the medical consultant explaining your actions and asking where you went wrong.

b.   Ignore the email as you were right and acted in line with family and your consultant.

c.   Inform the consultant with whom you discussed the case yesterday.

d.   Put in an incident report about the other consultant's behaviour.

e.   Inform your clinical supervisor.

f.   Ask an emergency registrar for advice.

g.   Decide not to do any further end of life discussions as an F1 per the medical consultant's email.

h.   Ask your friend on the medical ward who saw the patient in the morning why the medical consultant did not like your decision.

5.2 SJT Mock Answers

1.
Best answer: d
This avoids a scene and supports your colleague while gathering information before deciding on any action
Worst answer: b
Although you heard him shouting there may be many factors you are not aware of, escalating this, with limited information by confronting a consultant directly is unlikely to be a good choice as an F1
Middle answers: e, c, a
This question focuses on communication between yourself and your seniors, and maintaining a good level of professional communication. (d) Is the best option as it allows you to continue to inform the consultant of his duty towards patients, and therefore not compromise patient care, as well as later ascertaining how your colleague is feeling and help them resolve the situation. Immediately checking on your colleague (e) would help come to a resolution over the consultant's treatment of them, but may lead to a delay in the ward round and ultimately could compromise patient care. Informing your clinical supervisor (c) may facilitate a resolution to your colleague's problems, but it may also exacerbate the situation, as you have limited information as to the cause of the problem. Although this is better than ignoring the issue altogether (a), as it will not bring to light the potential mistreatment of junior staff. (b) Is the worst choice. Without knowing all the facts you may indirectly inflame the situation and lead to a further breakdown in professional communication.

2.
Best answer: a
Given their age, if they fulfil the criteria they can consent for treatment despite their parents
Worst answer: b
Although in their best interests it is not needed as they are able to consent and in doing the procedure without consent in someone able to do so, even with good intentions, it could be construed as assault
Middle answers: c, d, e
If a patient is under the age of 16, Gillick competence can be used to assess whether the patient is able to consent for a procedure without the permission of the parents. Therefore, this needs to be assessed (a), and is preferential to asking your registrar (c) straight away as they may be busy with other patients or in theatre. Discussing with the parents (d) may ascertain the reasons behind their refusal for surgery, but may not resolve the issue. However, this is preferable to informing the consultant (e), without attempting other avenues, as they are likely to be busy or not currently in the hospital (as it is an on-call shift). Performing the procedure without gaining consent (b), even if it is in the best interests of the patient, is not acceptable in this case as the patient is likely able to be consented for the procedure.

3.
Best Answer: A
Your first responsibility is to the patient and if they require surgery to have this in timely manner.
Worst Answer: D
This is completely inappropriate, if he cannot drive then it is unlikely he can operate.
Middle answers: B, C, E.
Rationale here is if no one if available to do it safely it should not happen until morning, C gets theatre ready to operate in the hope of minimizing a delay when a fit surgeon is found. E does not address any current issues and although not as bad as E is not helpful.

4.
Best answer A,
In the case of obstructive in patient teams and a sick patient this is likely to solve the situation fastest and optimize patient management
Worst answer B,
Clearly inappropriate as the patient is unwell
Middle order D, C, E.
D addresses the renal failure and high potassium but not the central issue, c may be helpful but the patient has other problems that even immediate urology input will not cure and is likely to need shared care or ITU. E although not as wrong as B does nothing for the patient.

5.
Best answer: D
You should always discuss these to allow the patient to be fully informed and to assess capacity
Worst answer: B
This would be inappropriate and cause the patient harm
Middle answers: E, C, A.
As an F1 who is not allowed to independently discharge patients involving a senior in a self-discharge situation would always be sensible to ensure you are not missing anything. C adds a witness to any decisions and an opinion which could be useful to your decision. A, although the patient may have metastasis if he is lucid and has capacity this would not change his ability to make decisions for which you have assessed him capable.

6.
Best answer: C
This is about confidentiality and you need the patients consent to give out any information
Worst answer: B
For the above reasons of confidentiality of your patient this is the worst answer, above being rude
Middle answers: E, D, A
Option E only defers the discussion but may buy you time to talk to the patient, D puts the onus on the patient but this may upset or distress her and is abdicat-

ing responsibility on your part. Putting the phone down is rude and is likely to aggravate any anger on the daughter's part.

7.
Best answer: D
You have never seen or done I&D before and should not be attempting one without senior support
Worst answer: A
This is not in the patients interests currently
Middle answers: E, C, B
Starting antibiotics is safe but unlikely to be of much benefit, it is better than doing a procedure you are not trained on either with a scalpel or a needle.

8.
Best answer: A
You can accept this and sharing it is the best option
Worst answer: C
There is no need to reject the gift that the family has given
Middle answers: B, E, D. It is better to share them with the team, e – throwing the gift away is unnecessary and will not gain anything. D – it is a low monetary gift and does not need to be declared

9.
Best answer: D
This escalates appropriately to your senior
Worst answer: C
You should not lie to your senior
Middle answers: E, B, A
The consultant is next to escalate too but you should follow the chain and ask your registrar first. This defers the issue but does not forget it, although it is not ideal as the team and family will want decisions to be made. Asking the surgical registrar for an opinion on a specialist field likely not to be his is unlikely to solve anything.

10.
Best answer: B
Always talk to the individual first to address the issue
Worst answer: E
This will not help anyone
Middle answers: A, D, C
Doing nothing leaves the issue unresolved, D could cause your colleague trouble unfairly if there is an innocent explanation you have not asked for, likewise with contacting the GMC.

11.
Best answer: B
You are not set up to have a breaking bad news conversation nor do you know the answer to many of its ramifications, it is much better to do this with a senior.
Worst answer: C

This will only cause concern and leave them to worry until tomorrow, although the scan says probable you may be wrong.

Middle answers: D, A, E

Having family present is helpful but also triggers concern for bad news, lying about your knowledge of the scan is not appropriate. Ignoring the patient although rude is better than C.

12.

Best answer: B

The patient should be seen but this is the most appropriate step if you are uncomfortable

Worst answer: A

This will not help and disadvantage your other patients as all of your patients will likely be cancelled and not be seen today.

Middle answers: E, D, C

Having your supervisor present could represent a learning opportunity for you and also means you are not alone with the patient. Seeing the patient if you are uncomfortable is not ideal and may compromise their care. Cancelling the appointment is worse as the patient may need to be seen urgently.

13.

Best answer: C

Having a frank discussion with daughter is likely to be most helpful and solve and misconceptions about end of life care

Worst answer: B

This would not help the situation or the patient

Middle answers: E, A, D

Discussing with your consultant may help if she continues to be concerned. Increasing the morphine PRNs may be a compromise and placate the daughter as the patient is comfortable and will not need them. There is no need to increase the diazepam at present, as the patient is not agitated.

14.

Best answer: E

Children under 18 can have things done in the patient's best interests if needed

Worst answer: A

He does not need to be consented under guardianship act as he can just be treated in best interests as he currently unwell enough to warrant this. The guardianship act also is more convoluted to invoke and is not used acutely often.

Middle answers: B, D, C

The parents do need to be contacted urgently, ideally they would be involved but if they cannot be reached then you can still proceed with surgery. Involving the teachers is probably good practice although not essential to a best interests consent.

15.

Best answer: C

This has clearly not been discussed with the daughter and she does not understand what it means

Worst answer: A

This is not appropriate and may lead to inappropriate CPR

Middle answers – D, B, E

Option D closely follows C, while B is unnecessarily antagonistic, E escalates to a senior who although busy will likely be able to deal with it well.

16.

Best answer: B

Your senior needs to review the patient if you feel they need surgery

Worst answer: A

This in an ineffective use of resources

Middle answers : E, D, C

Option E deals with the issue in clear order of priority, ignoring the call may delay important antibiotics while C neglects sick patient.

17.

Best answer: D

This will stop patient names being added and you can look up the other details using that

Worst answer: E

This will not help at this time

Middle answers: A, B, C

Attention to today's jobs comes first so checking the list is up to date is useful. Informing your educational supervisor may be helpful but no immediately, removing yourself from the group is likely to impact on patient care and create more work as you may miss additions to the list.

18.

Best answer: D

You are not allowed to do FP10s and so must find the quickest and safest way to have one issued.

Worst answer: A

You are working outside of your supervised practice and as such is not safe and not allowed.

Middle answers: B, E, C

This is a commonly occurring issue in real practice, and certainly one not often explained properly at medical school.

FP10 prescriptions are outpatient prescription for use in community pharmacies. These prescriptions can be used by hospital doctors in limited circumstances – e.g. analgesia or antibiotics - as most things can wait until next GP appointment. F1s are only supposed to prescribe medication as part of their education, and ultimately what they prescribe is the responsibility of supervisors, therefore F1s are not allowed to prescribe on FP10 forms, or dispense medication alone. In this case there is a patient who requires medication, and needs to be discharged. Whilst E is correct, it does not solve the issue of the patient requiring discharge, therefore D is likely the best answer, as the surgical SHO is able to complete an FP10. B is still better than E, as it expedites the discharge, but you will be interrupting the SpR in theatre, and they certainly will not be able to sign

MOCK SJT

anything until they have de-scrubbed!
Of options A & C- C is the better answer as although the SpR will almost certainly tell you the correct medication & doses these may not be in line with local guidelines.

19.
Best answer: C
This provides a sick patient in need of escalation the quickest and best care by senior staff in the hospital.
Worst answer: E
Prescribing a drug you are not familiar with based on an indication you do not know is not safe.
Middle answer: D, A, B

This question focuses on a couple of issues, though the bottom line is you are no longer in a position to manage this patient on your own.GMC guidance is clear on prescribing, and particularly with regards to F1s it states that you should only prescribe within the limits of your competence. In addition, this patient is deteriorating which makes any decisions more time pressured. The ideal course of action would be to discuss the case with the medical registrar on call, however they have not replied to you in this scenario (most likely as they are with another unwell patient).
Ultimately, if you are out of you comfort zone with a rapidly deteriorating patient, the safest course of action is to put out a peri-arrest / medical emergency call (C), and you will rapidly receive support. Alternatively speaking to another senior such as the F2, (D) or SHO for advice is a sensible option if the patient is stable enough, as they will likely be able to come and help you. Bleeping the medical registrar again is a possibility as even though they may not answer they will be aware that your call is urgent
B is an excellent idea for you learning but not a great idea if you are sitting in front of an acutely unwell patient. Likewise, E is not safe as discussed above, as there may be countless reasons this treatment is not suitable or may even be unsafe for this patient.

20.
Best Answer: D
This is a potential never event and the relevant proof needs to be found quickly and ideally with as little offence as possible.
Worst answer: B
This ignores any concerns and allows wrong site surgery to occur, potentially making you culpable too.
Middle answers: C, A, E
This is a real case, and happened in Wales in 2000. It was a medical student, not an F1 who pointed out it was the wrong kidney, and they were ignored by the consultant and SpR. The patient died and the both surgeons were charged with manslaughter.
Wrong site surgery itself is a "never event", i.e. A preventable error with potentially serious consequences for the patient.In this case clearly if you have concern you cannot let the surgery proceed. Presumably the only reason the

medical student was not prosecuted as well was because she had raised a concern. If the consultant is unwilling to listen to you, it is best to provide some evidence (D) that he is making a mistake. If this fails the next best option is to try another route by talking to the anaesthetist (C). Option A is clearly very confrontational, but may be a sensible "last resort" if you are not left with any other options, though clearly would require a lot of bravery to do in real life!
Options B & E are clearly the worst as they allow the surgery to proceed, but at least with E you are raising your concerns a second time.

21.
Best Answer: C
This protects you, maintaining professionalism while ensuring patient care is not compromised.
Worst Answer: D
As tempting as this may be, it is not safe.
Middle answers: B, E, A

Complaints are sadly an inevitable part of a career in medicine, and it is important to be aware of this. If you do end up in a situation like this, it is important to reflect on the issues, and get support – a sensible first point of call would be your educational supervisor.
From the information above, it does appear the patient is behaving unreasonably, but all complaints must be taken seriously, as poor handling of the complaint, particularly initially may lead to unnecessary escalation and or litigation. With all complaints, you need to continue to provide a good standard of care for patients. Good medical practice states:"61. You must respond promptly, fully and honestly to complaints and apologise when appropriate. You must not allow a patient's complaint to adversely affect the care or treatment you provide or arrange.
62. You should end a professional relationship with a patient only when the breakdown of trust between you and the patient means you cannot provide good clinical care to the patient."
From this clearly A&D are the least appropriate actions, as it results in a substandard provision of care for the patient, with D the worst option as the patient would not be seen at all. It does not appear form the question that "the breakdown of trust means you cannot provide a good standard of care" as per the GMC guidelines, though it may progress to this in the future.
E provides a safe option for the patient, but it may be sensible to protect yourself. Therefore, B is a better option, but again the SHO may not be in every day, and may need to see the more unwell patients on the ward. Therefore, C is the best option, as the patient receives a regular review, and having a chaperone as a witness may reassure yourself and the patient.

22.
Best answer: D
As with many things in medicine you often will never improve without trying and will often surprise yourself when you do. Difficulty is not an excuse in this case to avoid the task. Your requests for help will usually be better received if you have tried yourself.

Worst answer: E
Missed antibiotics are likely to have an adverse outcome on the patient's care.
Middle answers: A, B, C
This is a frequently occurring problem out of hours. Antibiotic levels are important, as levels may be sub-therapeutic or toxic. They also need taking at specific times; therefore, it is not acceptable to do nothing (E), as this may endanger patient safety.
The best solution is to attempt to take a sample yourself (D), and you should not really proceed with any of the other options until you have at least had an attempt. The next best option would be to ask your SHO and then to take an arterial sample, though it would be best practice to attempt a venous sample first. You could ask the anaesthetist on ward cover as a last resort (C).

23.
Best answer: B
Where possible especially when in extremis like this you should attempt to involve next of kin in all end of life decisions.
Worst answer: A
This borders on potential misleading of the family and without a clear plan to communicate this later there is potential for it to be missed completely.
Middle answers: C, D, E

The guidance on this has recently changed following a high court judgment. The ruling stated that DNACPR decisions should be discussed with patients before the decision is made, "provided it is appropriate and practical to do so."
The actual case involved a DNACR decision that was not discussed with the mother of a patient overnight. She took the clinicians to court not over the decision, but with the fact it was not discussed with her. Clearly this is not a decision you will be involved in alone as an F1, but an awareness of the ethics involved is necessary as you progress through your training.
In this scenario, the best course is to discuss with the family before signing the form (B), although it should be noted the DNACPR is a clinical decision that has already been made, so C is the next best answer.As the patient is deteriorating, it is likely that by morning it would be too late to discuss with the family, though in option D at least the form had been completed and the patient will not receive unnecessary and likely futile CPR.
Option E is preferable to option A, as at least the family will be informed, though as the patient is deteriorating overnight again, this discussion may not wait until morning.

24.
Best answer: c
The best option here is to explore the patient's feelings and if possible avoid a complaint being made by satisfying the patient that such behaviour will not be tolerated
Worst answer: d
The worst answer here is to lie to the patient
Middle answers: b, e, a
There may be other factors behind the patient's complaint so having the senior

nurse there may help address these and give you some support in a potentially difficult scenario. While apologising (b) is never a bad idea it does little to remedy the underlying complaint and makes no effort to stop a potentially avoidable complaint. Asking the Middle grade doctor (e) may seem like a direct solution however it could be potentially embarrassing for the doctor in question and if they are defensive it could lead to a confrontational scenario with the patient, which may only make matters worse. Belittling the patient's complaint (a) is only going to make matters worse.

25.
Best answer: d
Communicating directly with your colleague allows you to raise the issue without embarrassing them and explore any issues that colleague may have, e.g.: it may be that the ward soap irritates their skin.
Worst answer: e
This doesn't directly address your concern about patient safety, doesn't explore your colleague's point of view and shows a complete lack of team communication.
Middle answers: b, c, a
If you discuss with your colleague in a sensitive and honest way you are unlikely to damage your working relationship but asking another colleague (b) to do so is an option, although it abdicates your responsibility somewhat and is not the job of the Senior Nurse, although he/she may be happy to oblige. Undertaking an infection control audit (c) gives you an opportunity to educate the whole team and raise standards across the ward however it is an indirect and time-consuming method of remedying the issue when you have only noticed one colleague at fault. It may still be a better option than embarrassing your colleague in front of the entire team (a) and possibly irreparably damaging your work relationship.

26.
Best answer: d
While a commitment to medical education is admirable we must ensure that patient confidentiality is not breached. The best thing to do if you are unsure is to ask advice. They would most likely refer you to GMC guidance on Social Media use by doctors which has information and practical advice for such situations.
Worst answer: c
You cannot blindly accept your colleagues' assurances. Unfortunately, no social media site can guarantee privacy despite your settings and once you share patient identifiable details you cannot control the extent to which they are shared further on other social media platforms.
Middle answers: b, e, a
If after discussion with the colleague in question you do not feel that your concerns have been addressed then it is appropriate to speak to someone with managerial or pastoral responsibility for that trainee (b). Canvassing opinion (e) may lead to you getting the right advice however it may also mislead you and has the disadvantage of involving lots of people in a potentially embarrassing situation which may result in disciplinary procedures. Your colleague will not thank you for getting the whole staff gossiping about her. By leaving the group and pursuing the matter no further (a) you are doing nothing to ensure that

patient confidentiality is protected in future. All the above options are preferable to (c).

27.
Best answer: a
Spending time exploring your colleague's concerns (1) and giving them a confidence boost from another perspective will likely be therapeutic in its own right and shouldn't be overlooked given its simplicity to perform.
Worst Answer: d
Asking other team members to take on more work (4) is unfair on them, does not tackle the underlying issue and lets more people in on an issue which your colleague told you in confidence.
Middle answers: c, e, b
Recommending they speak to a supervisor with a pastoral role (C) is appropriate as the trainee's health may be at risk. This would be a more appropriate choice than you speaking to a different senior doctor without that trainee present (E) especially as there have been no concerns raised about the doctor's performance on that firm. Offering to cover shifts (B) is a nice gesture however you should not put yourself in a position where you are over-worked without proper time to recover. The temporary relief does not affect the underlying issue and the anxiety may return once again. Asking other team members to take on more work (4) is unfair on them, does not tackle the underlying issue and lets more people in on an issue which your colleague told you in confidence.

28.
Best Answer: e
If you are not satisfied that your concerns have been properly listened to then you should try another avenue. In this case as it is a clinical matter pertaining to the day-to-day workings of the practice it would be more appropriate to discuss with a senior partner
Worst answer: c
Continuing in a role that you believe is beyond your competency is a risk to patient safety and should be avoided at all costs.
Middle answers: d, b, a
Speaking to your educational supervisor (d) who is likely a specialist in a different field is less beneficial than speaking to a partner in the practice. Your educational supervisor is more concerned with a pastoral and educational role – although they are of course a good source of advice and support should you need it. Restricting your role to seeing simpler patients (b) has the advantage of continuing to help out the practice with their workload and ensure patients are reviewed in a timely fashion however it limits your educational development, and there is still potential for misjudgement of the severity of a condition over the phone leaving you out of your depth. Refusing to perform the duty (a) will jeopardise your working relationship with your supervisor and an inability to negotiate with colleagues and communicate properly. It will often only inflame the situation rather than resolve it and takes the focus off your valid concerns.

29.
Best answer: d

As always tackling the issue directly with the person involved is the best approach as long as you can raise the issue tactfully.

Worst answer: a

While a colleague's personal life is their own, when it has the potential to adversely impact on both their and patient safety, then you do have a duty to intervene.

Middle answers: b, e, c

If you are concerned that such a conversation between peers would be difficult then discreetly asking an appropriate senior doctor (b) to help you is appropriate. Trying to avoid embarrassing a colleague (e) is an admirable motivation but you are not tackling the issue directly. Keeping a tally (c) is a wholly useless thing to do without taking action and potentially heading off a dangerous situation.

30.

Best answer: e

Everyone makes mistakes and as a junior doctor you are not immune to this. Senior doctors know this and will learn more about you by how you react than the fact that you made them. Being honest, admitting your mistake and suggesting a possible solution shows your integrity and dedication.

Worst answer: b

Being dishonest should always be avoided.

Middle answers: c, a ,d

Attempts to remedy the situation should be made if feasible (c) but shouldn't be done as a way to cover-up a mistake. Asking the nurses to help (a) may be tempting but they have their own duties and shouldn't be put under pressure with extra jobs as they prepare for the ward round as well. The last two options do nothing to remedy the situation and see you attempt to shift blame elsewhere. If you have genuine concerns about your workload (d) you should have raised them earlier and to do so now seems petulant and disingenuous.

31.

Best answer: b

Your intentions in helping your colleague were admirable but it has begun to impact on your training. A consultant has noticed this and your route now should be open and honest.

Worst answer: d

Suggesting that the Trust needs to employ a locum (4) to make life easier for your colleague is dishonest and wasteful as you had been able to cover your half of the work without trouble.

Middle answers: a, c, e

Your colleague will not get the help they require if you continue to cover for them (a) and this will likely negatively impact on both of you despite your best efforts. In all but the first option you are not being completely honest with your supervisor but (a) is superior to (c) in so far as the running of the ward and by extension, patient safety, is not compromised by a decision to work to rule. Maintaining the status quo (e) where your colleague doesn't get the support they need and your training continues to suffer is a poor option. Any concerns about a trainee need to be identified early to ensure patient safety and that the trainee is supported before things get worse.

32.
Best answer: a
This issue needs to be tackled directly and this is the only option that does so.
If the two senior members of a team are working at cross-purposes then the
team will not function effectively with a potential impact on patient care.
Worst answer: c
Disobeying the direct instructions of your consultant without letting them know
directly gains nothings and undermines the consultant who is ultimately responsible.
Middle answers: e, b, d
If resolution between the consultant and registrar cannot be done, then the
consultant retains overall responsibility for the patient's care under their name
hence their plans should be followed (e). Asking a different senior doctor (b)
may ensure patient safety is protected and they may take a lead in resolving this
conflict but this is not their role and it puts them in an awkward situation; never
mind asking them to make decisions about patients who are not under their
care. Option (d) is likely to give the appearance of telling tales and will likely only
stir up conflict in your team even further.

33.
Best answer: e
This question explores your dedication to patient focus and your communication
skills. The best approach here is to attempt to discuss the patient's concerns
directly. It is important that you can empathise with a patient and it is likely that if
you spend time understanding a patient's viewpoint then you will find a solution.
Worst answer: d
The worst option here is to ignore the patient and do the operation yourself by
withholding the patient's wishes from the rest of the team.
Middle answers: b, c, a
Asking you consultant to do this is another option (b) and their presence may
carry more gravitas for this particular patient but it takes the consultant away
from other commitments and misses the opportunity for you to develop your
communication skills. If no compromise or solution can be reached then the
patient's wishes should be respected (c) as long as it is appropriate to do so.
Option (a) is confrontational and unhelpful. Of course, patients should have
input into their care and using the delay of their care as a threat is highly inappropriate.

34.
Best answer: c
As important as antibiotics are, a short delay is unlikely to change much and if
the ward round is just you and the consultant, not seeing the other patients or
delaying their review is likely to be worse
Worst answer: e
This would be a waste of time trying to place blame and achieves nothing
Middle answers: b, a, d
In the first instance, you should seek the advice of your consultant (c). It may

be that you can be spared from the round to insert the cannula and if not then your consultant can make an alternative plan for the antibiotics to be delivered. Dosage schedules of antibiotics are important to provide an appropriate and constant level of therapy (b) however you should not abandon the ward round without discussing with your consultant first. Maintaining a professional relationship with all the team is important for safe and effective practice (a), it may fall to you to rise about rude behaviour and address the situation to maintain cordiality however it is not an urgent consideration. The patient's notes should not be used for tit-for-tat pettiness, the facts of patient's care such as the insertion of cannulas or the reason for delay in antibiotic administration should be entered (d). Wasting your time in enquiries which will not change the present situation should not be high on the list of your priorities (e).

35.
Best answer: d
Dealing with the situation immediately and personally is always going to be the quickest route to the answer
Worst answer: e
Doing nothing is clearly the worst answer
Middle answers: a, b, c
The most appropriate and compassionate answer is to speak directly to your colleague and gather information (d). You do not know what is being discussed behind closed doors but likely your colleague will see your concern as genuine and respond well to it. Bluntly advising them to see a counsellor (a) makes no attempt at understanding their situation but does show your concern whereas option (b) doesn't even do that. They do have the benefit of speaking directly to your colleague whereas going immediately over their head to their supervisor (c) will damage your professional relationship without making any attempt to speak to the person or clarify the situation. It would become a more appropriate option if you had already attempted to make a direct intervention and were concerned it had made no difference. Burying your head in the sand and taking no action (e) is an abdication of your responsibility to your co-workers and shows a failure to communicate effectively.

36.
Best answer: a
The alternative is lying which is you are not allowed to do, this is the truth which is what is expected
Worst answer: d
This is a clear lie and that makes it the worst answer
Middle answers: c, e, b
Uncomfortable as it may be, if you are asked a direct question by your consultant it is imperative that you do not lie (a). Professional integrity is essential as a doctor and your colleague should know he has put you in an impossible situation. Asking your consultant to find out for themselves (c) is a way of avoiding telling the truth yourself. An understaffed ward is a danger to patient safety so your intentions are correct however you have simply avoided the question and it is unlikely to satisfy your consultant. Telling a lie either by omission (b) or directly (d) should be your least appropriate answers; by embellishing further

details one is slightly worse than the other.

37.
Best answer: e
Without knowing the patient's wishes about his information, you cannot disclose it
Worst answer: b
This could well be a severe breach of confidentiality
Middle answers: d, a, c
You cannot assume Mr Munroe is happy for his daughter-in-law or any family member to know his medical details. For that reason, it is best to politely decline her suggestion (e) whilst arranging a suitable time to pass the information on so that Mr Munroe does not become impatient or worried when he awakes. The on-call doctor may be able to come and have a chat with Mr Munroe (d) but this is less suitable as they will likely be busy and should prioritise urgent clinical duties and may not be familiar with Mr Munroe's case. Waking Mr Munroe up whilst he is sleeping (a) allows you to directly relay the information but whilst he is recuperating it is better to let him rest. A sealed envelope (c) may make an attempt at preserving confidentiality but it is hardly fool-proof and without an interpretation of the results or what it means for his on-going care Mr Munroe could become confused and anxious. However in this instance the breaking patient confidentiality (b) is the worst outcome.

38.
Best answer: b
You should not prescribe blindly without advice given you know this to be a very large and potentially inappropriate dose
Worst answer: a
Given what you know this could be dangerous, any ill effects would be your responsibility as the prescriber
Middle answer: d, c, e
The most appropriate action is to gather advice from an on-call senior colleague(b), their experience and guidance will hopefully lead to a safe and effective resolution to the problem. Gathering more information from experienced nursing staff (d) is a simple and appropriate thing to do however they are unlikely to be able to guide you in the same way as a senior registrar. They may at least have familiarity with giving a sedative dose of that amount which can indicate whether this is a prescription error or not. Going by the BNF recommended dose (c) is a safe and reasonable thing to do in uncertainty however it runs the risk of under-treating the patient and you have not made any attempt to find out why the consultant has recommended that dose. Waking your FY2 up overnight to ask a clinical question (e) is inappropriate and they will not thank you. On call senior cover is there for a reason and should be used. All these options are preferable to blindly prescribing what could be a transcription error without first investigating its appropriateness (a). It represents a risk to patient safety and as such should be avoided.

39.
Best answer: d

Raising the issue with the Registrar who may be stressed and not appreciate his own behaviour unless questioned in a non-confrontational manner. You then follow this up with your supervisor to de-brief on how it affected you and hope further action is taken to avoid the Registrar doing the same in the future.

Worst answer: c
Bullying should not be tolerated; neither have you reflected on the negative experience nor raised a concern to stop similar future events.

Middle answers: e, a, b
(e) is the next best as you actively debrief and pursue further action but less optimal than D as you do not try to resolve the issue with the person in question. (b) is the second worst as though trying to address the issue, you do so in a confrontational manner which is not professional leaving (a) the third option as you address the matter but no long-term action is taken to facilitate change.

40.
Best answer: a
Seeking to do the lumbar puncture under supervision is the best thing to do, you are unable to do it unsupervised but it is still a learning opportunity for you, without compromising patient safety.

Worst answer: b
Patient safety is paramount therefore doing the procedure with no immediate supervision to take over in the event something goes wrong is dangerous.

Middle answers: d, e, c
Seeking to do the lumbar puncture under supervision (a) is better than just observing it (d) as you have previously observed two; observing another one will not further your learning whereas performance under supervision will. (e) is more optimal than (c) as you actively seek and offer a solution rather than merely refusing to do the lumbar puncture.

41.
Best answer: d
D is the best option as you point Dorothy in the direction of feedback which will be encouraging and help improve services while not taking the money which is more productive than just refusing to take the money.

Worst answer: c
Accepting the money would be unprofessional and go against GMC advice for large gifts unless you declare it.

Middle answers: a, e, b
Accepting the money is unprofessional however (b) is slightly better then (c) as you share it with colleagues for communal good. (a) is more appropriate than (e) as the latter suggests you are still trying to claim the money but just refusing to by word.

42.
Best answer: d
This is the only option that deals with the problem immediately protecting patients and thus the most appropriate first.

Worst answer: e
As this may be a breech of confidentiality, offering to help is by no means ap-

MOCK SJT

propriate and the worst answer from this scenario.

Middle answers: a, b, c

This scenario brings into question patient confidentiality, social media and communicating with colleagues. (a) is the next most appropriate as he may not appreciate the severity of his actions therefore bringing this to his attention would be necessary. (b) is more appropriate than (c) as you he will need supervision and support from a senior regarding a very complicated matter and you as an FY1 will not be in the best position to advice on consent or ethical approval with limited research experience yourself.

43.

Best answer: e

This addresses the issue as you take a proactive role in crating a solution. Although coming in before your start time is not ideal or a long-term solution, this is temporary and sharing the work load before a solution can be made with senior advice.

Worst answer: b

Refusing to continue without finding a solution is no solution at all and would be irresponsible and compromise the team as well as the patients.

Middle answers: d, c, a

(c & d) work on the process of escalation if your thoughts are not acknowledged and acted upon. Talking to your clinical supervisor (d) is more likely to have a lasting change than discussing with your FY1 colleagues (c). Continuing to do the lists without mentioning your concerns, though kind, is not a fair solution (a) but better than just refusing as mentioned previously (b). Trainees should be able to freely express their thoughts in their posts.

44.

Best answer: d

This answer addresses your professional commitment in the politest way to the patient

Worst answer: b

By doing this it encourages further blurring of the lines between your personal and professional life

Middle answers: a, e, c

It is against GMC guidance to befriend patients to whom you are in a position of trust as a doctor. As such (c & b) would be inappropriate and (b) is more inappropriate as (c) ensures you are not friends on social media long term – therefore dealing with the problem although in a deceiving way. (d & a) actively deal with the problem instead of just ignoring it (e). (d) is more appropriate as you explain in honesty why it would not be appropriate whereas refuting a patient for what they may see as a gesture of kindness will have a lasting negative impact on your relationship with the patient (a).

45.

Best answer: b

Your own safety and that of other staff comes first so calling security is appropriate as a first step closely followed by verbal de-escalation

Worst answer: c
This does not deal with the problem at hand
Middle answers: a, e, d
As the patient has threatened to physically abuse staff, you must call security immediately (b). While they get to you it will be worthwhile using de-escalation methods to diffuse the situation (a). Medical sedation should be seen as a last resort and avoided where possible but in this case may be appropriate (e). Rehydrating Eleanor and referral to substance misuse are both reasonable but do not need to be done in the immediate situation you are faced with; (d) being more pressing than (c) as the liaison psychiatry team will often be busy seeing other patients.

46.
Best answer: b
Preventing any potential drug error is the priority
Worst answer: a
Although not wrong this is the least immediate answer and importantly not harm had occurred but it was a potential near miss
Middle answers: c, d, e
This question is all about patient safety. The task of ensuring the patient does not receive the incorrect medicine is paramount. As such (b & c) are the most pressing tasks (b) more so as the nurse may have drawn up the drug to administer prior to documenting it has been administered. (d) is the next most pressing task as it corrects the mistake made ensuring the patient gets the right medication. (e) goes about addressing the mistake to avoid it occurring again but has no impact on this patient. Finally, a serious incident form should be filled for this near miss but is not an immediate priority (a).

47.
Best answers: b, g, h
Eliminate clearly wrong: d, e
This question has fewer clearly wrong options and so is harder but these are of no help to resolving the situation. The key to the question is removing the confidential information from the public domain as quickly as possible. G is the best answer as it solves with problem quicker, B also addresses the problem but probably slower. H is part of a duty of candour and although embarrassing is better than being caught and not having declared it. E and D are possibly valid but is likely to be a mistake so may be excessive and also does nothing to remove the photo. The other options all do not address the issue directly or quickly enough.

48.
Best answers: d, f, h
Eliminate clearly wrong: c, e
This question deals with patient safety in emotive circumstances and issues such as these with staffing are not uncommon. D is obviously the best answer as it is safe an enables you to go, F is far from ideal but may represent a compromise ensuring the evening on call is covered. H is not ideal either but if the alternative is an unfilled on call this could seriously affect patient safety.

A, B and H may help but are unlikely to be quick or successful in time to help your cause given your consultant and medical staffing are already involved. C is obviously dishonest and unsafe.

49.
Best answers: c, e, a
Eliminate clearly wrong: d, h
This question is about dealing with conflict and difficult individuals at work, it is also deliberately difficult and most answers are not ideal. C cuts to the root cause and may help solve the issue. E is also helpful as your clinical supervisor will work in the department and know the individual and be better placed the address the issue. Given the other options A is next best as you are still asking seniors for help but where possible suggesting if no one else was free you would still ask for help and not make decisions on your own. B does nothing to address the issue, D is too rash as although harsh in his words he may have a point and many more "old school" consultants do teach in this way. F would be unsafe, G does nothing to solve the issue and H would involve a lot of work on your part and potentially clashing runs of shift just to avoid an individual.

50.
Best answers: a, e, h
Eliminate clearly wrong: c, d
Both of these avoid dealing with the issue at heart and crucially break your colleagues trust.
As with most questions on the SJT, the most important issue is patient safety. Whilst it does not appear to have had any effect on patient safety thus far there is clearly the potential.
Regardless of her decisions with the pregnancy, it is probably sensible for her to speak to her GP, particularly as it is impacting on her health and ability to practice safely at present.Educational supervisors are the first port of call for welfare issues. It would be a good idea for her to discuss with hers for further advice and support. In this vein if you are struggling with your responsibilities (i.e. keeping the list up to date) as a result it would be sensible to speak to your educational supervisor. A solution might be to involve the F2 or SHO, but this does not solve any of the issues with regards to your fellow F1 who is clearly in need of some support.

51.
Best answers: c, f, h
Eliminate clearly wrong: b, d, e
None of these options address the problem in hand and most are to your detriment so are wrong.
A - may provide some helpful tips, though remember these are also new F1s and may be struggling too.B – as attractive as an option this is, F1 teaching attendance is a requirement of passing the foundation programme.
C – Very sensible, particularly if they are finishing on time every day and you are not. They may also be able to advise which of the jobs can be delegated to others, or are less urgent and can be delayed.D – whilst this may have an element of truth, it is not a helpful way to think, and does not solve any problems. Maybe

the current staffing levels are inappropriate and need addressing? Ignoring the problems will mean they continue for the next F1s who replace you.

E- same as DF- sensible option, Educational supervisors are first point of call if you are struggling

G – whilst may be a good idea to discuss with your consultant, it would be more appropriate to do this in private rather than interrupting a ward round.H- Yes. Your clinical supervisor is a consultant in the specialty you are working in, so would also be a good person to speak to.

52.
Best answers: d, f, g
Eliminate clearly wrong: e, h
Both of these are clearly wrong as you are competent to do neither and a nurse chaperone makes no difference.

A- Technically correct, but not ideal, you are missing al earning opportunity.

B- As above

C- This would be correct if you have seen one before, but is unsafe if you have not previously observed the procedure

D- Correct, the procedure will be performed safely and it provides a good opportunity for you to learn more about the procedure

E- Unsafe, since you have not performed the procedure before

F- A good idea, and will help you explain the procedure to the patient before it is performed

G- A good idea, and polite if you ask someone else to do a procedure for you

H- Great if you are able to, but since you have not seen the procedure before and are therefore unlikely to have an in-depth knowledge of it this would not be valid consent

53.
Best answers: b, e, h
Eliminate clearly wrong: d, f
Both of these have no immediate action and put the onus on someone else to follow up a potentially serious diagnosis of which you cannot be sure will be done.

Whilst unfortunate, this is a scenario that does happen, and it is often left to foundation doctors to follow up on histological samples, as the result if often not received for some weeks after the specimen is sent.

Clearly the patient needs to be informed of this, though you would not be in a position to do so, as you have not met the patient before, therefore A would be inappropriate.The patient's GP needs to be informed (B), but as the test was arranged in secondary care it is the responsibility of the hospital team to act on any results – not the responsibility of the GP, so F is inappropriate.

The patient will need follow up at the hospital – this is best done by the consultant and local cancer specialist services (E & H).Whilst it is a good idea to inform the consultant, email is not a reliable method of communication, particularly as this is your last day of F1 (And potentially last at the trust); therefore C is incorrect.

The surgical registrar is a good person to speak to for advice, and may be able to point you in the right direction, but you should arrange follow up as above rather than simply handing over for the registrar to arrange. Clearly the new staring F1s will have more to worry about than tying up your loose ends (G&D).

54.
Best answers: c, d, h
Eliminate clearly wrong: b, e, g
The key problem with all three is that you are not allowed to prescribe chemotherapy and as such all are wrong even with best intentions.

F1s should only prescribe things they have a knowledge of when it is safe and they are confident to do so. F1s are not allowed to prescribe chemotherapy. If fact, chemotherapy decisions should be undertaken by a specialist. Chemotherapy decisions are tailored to each patient, and have the potential for severe adverse effects, particularly if prescribed incorrectly. Therefore B,E,F and G are incorrect.
Option A is a good idea, but this could certainly wait until morning (D).
The patient may require some of their other medicines and analgesia, which you could prescribe (C), though it would be important to document clearly on the chart and in the notes that you had created a duplicate drug chart.
Clearly the drug chart needs to be found, and the issue may be resolved quickly if you are able to help the nurses find the missing chart (H).

55.
Best answers: c, d, g
Eliminate as clearly wrong: a, b, e, f
It is against GMC guidance for a doctor to 'date' a patient as it could be an abuse of power given that patients are in vulnerable states when in hospitals. As such, options (a, e, f and h) are inappropriate. Of the remaining options, (c, d & g) are far less confrontational than (b) with the same outcome of not going out.

56.
Best answer: a, e, h
Eliminate as clearly wrong: b, c, d, g
The main issues addressed here are that of patient safety, consent and competence. Though you have assisted in the procedure once, it is a complicated operation with significant risks and as such you should not be consenting the patient as a foundation trainee (b, f and g). (d) is unacceptable as you would be lying and creating an unnecessary and unexpected delay by not warning the registrar and consultant you will not consent the patient. The other four options are all acceptable but whereas in (b) you just refuse to consent the patient, in (a, e & h) you are seeking active means by which to aid the process of consenting the patient without risking their safety. (c) does not provide a solution to the consenting issue unlike the three best answers.

57.
Best answers: b, d, e

Eliminate as clearly wrong: a, c, g, h
GMC guidance advises that clinicians should avoid treating family, friends and patients whom they know to reduce the impairment of clinical judgment which may be caused by this. Given that they have made their intentions clear to the nurse, you can rest knowing they are GCS 15 and well enough to speak therefore there is no matter of urgent clinical need. As such, seeing him would not be appropriate (a & f). Equally avoiding seeing him without handing over to a colleague would be unprofessional (g). Calling security (c) or completing an incident form (h) are both extreme and inappropriate as he has not done anything warranting such action. The correct answer would be to ask the nurse to relay information that he will be seen when appropriate, that you are currently busy and hand over his case to a colleague (b, d, e).

58.
Best Answers: c, d, f
Eliminate as clearly wrong: a, b, g
Though the patient is not directly under your care, as a doctor it is your duty to care for patients in need. As such refusing to prescribe is completely unacceptable and goes against your duties as a doctor (a & b). You should offer to prescribe analgesia (c) and even assess her quickly (d) to see if this is a gynae emergency requiring immediate care and moving to resus while the gynae team come to assess. In light of this and the fact the nurses have tried to contact gynae for an hour with no response, escalation is an appropriate step of action (f). Bleeping the gynae SHO will be no different to what the nurses have been doing for an hour and will unlikely have a different outcome (e). Asking the surgical team to come and would be an inappropriate referral as a GP has sent her for gynae assessment (g). (h) would not be particularly useful as she will still need to be seen by gynae and you should be able to assess whether this appears to by a gynae emergency.

59.
Best answers: f, g, h
Eliminate as clearly wrong: a, b, c, d, e
As a doctor, you have a duty of candour hence apologizing to the family would be completely appropriate despite not being directly involved (f). It would also be appropriate to give the family details of the PALS team (g) as they were clearly upset and may want to make a formal complaint. In addition, the issue will need to be addressed with the nurses directly (h) and you may need to speak to the ward sister as a matter of escalation. Ignoring the incident (a) or refuting the nurses in front of the family (b) would be inappropriate. (c) is a very passive approach to dealing with the problem and will be unlikely to be successful. Your educational supervisor (d) is not involved and this is not under their remit. Finally, option (e) would not be appropriate as the family were the ones affected and therefore the matter should be addressed with them (f & g).

60.
Eliminate clearly wrong: a, c, d, e, g
These options do nothing to help the situation and may be dangerous
Best answers: c, f, h

This question looks at your commitment to team working and your ability to recognise and integrate the concerns of co-workers such as nurses and allied health professionals. If there is dispute within the team about a patient's care then the best approach will be to get all parties in one room and discuss it (c). That is by far most likely to lead to a joint solution which everyone is happy with. At this meeting or another time, you should explore all party's viewpoints including your own (f) while bearing in mind that the medical angle is not necessarily the most important or relevant at that stage. While the physiotherapists are busy and might not appreciate their judgement being questioned, if you can politely request another review (h) then it may either validate the nurse's concerns or provide them the reassurance they need to allow Mrs Atkinson to begin mobilising independently. Other options where you dismiss the nurses' opinion (b) (e), attempt to circumvent their concerns without addressing the issue (d) (g) or just blindly accept one viewpoint in order to avoid conflict (a) are not appropriate.

61.
Eliminate clearly wrong: e, b
These do nothing to fix the situation and may jeopardise yours
Best answers: c, d, f
It is likely the doctor is already familiar with existing policy on accepting gifts from patients but has feels compelled to ignore them by his personal situation. That said it is still preferable to take a non-confrontational approach and re-affirm why exactly patient gifts are not accepted (c) rather than charge in with moral outrage (a). This is a personal issue but one that has the potential to impair his fitness to practice therefore it should be escalated to a senior doctor with a pastoral role (d). The CAB offer impartial advice on issues such as debt (f) and is a better solution than you becoming financially involved however good your intentions as it will only muddy your professional relationship (b). Options (e) and (g) are not in keeping with the GMC guidance on accepting gifts from patients. Option (h) does not directly address the issue.

62.
Eliminate clearly wrong: b, e
As per usual this does nothing to address the issue and so is wrong
Best answers: d, f, h
This scenario tests your communication, your team-working, your self-awareness and your character! It is never easy to hear criticism but it is how we react that determines our future performance. Accepting that your colleague has come to you in good faith to try and remedy the situation you should hear out the concerns and attempt to explore how you can learn from them (d). There are plenty of potential sources of support here including your supervisors (h) and peers who are setting a good example (e). There is no shame in addressing weaknesses in our development and no-one expects you to be a perfect doctor overnight, only to be willing to learn. Hence why being dismissive (b) or rude (e) are clearly wrong. A token gesture (c) will not change the underlying situation and going to far the other way is inappropriate – it is not a nurse's job to oversee doctor's plans and it shows an inability to understand their concerns (g). Asking for names so you can perform personal confrontations (a) is obviously not correct. They have gone to the nurse in charge specifically to avoid such an ugly

scenario.

63.
Eliminate clearly wrong: c, d, h
These would clearly antagonise the situation or attempt to shift the blame
Best answers: b, e, f
It is important to make a measured response to this situation. If you can empathise with the patient and her family then you will understand their frustration which has unfortunately led to one of them lashing out. Keeping your cool and apologising to de-escalate the situation will hopefully go a long way (e) towards calming them down and letting them see you care. Reminding them of hospital policy on aggression towards staff may be a next step if the situation remains tense (f), it is preferable to using security staff as a threat (c) although they may need to be called if the situation escalates further. Calling for the support of a senior doctor is appropriate (b), they will likely have more experience of this type of situation and can add support to your position. You should avoid making promises you cannot keep as this will only lead to future confrontations (a). Blaming the rehabilitation hospital is unhelpful and unprofessional, the relatives will likely not be impressed by this either (d). If the family request details of the complaints procedure then you should provide this however attempts should be made to remedy the situation before you offer it as a solution (g). Asking the nurses to get involved in a confrontational manner is not appropriate and risks worsening the situation considerably (h).

64.
Eliminate clearly wrong: c, f, g
These do nothing to directly address the situation
Best answers: b, e, h
One must always be aware of the difference in perspective between seasoned healthcare professionals who deal with such situations on a regular basis and a patient who is likely anxious and scared as their (or their babies) health is on the line. The situation itself along with the unfamiliar environment can be very distressing as care and compassion must be shown in order to minimise this as much as possible. Good communication with the mother, asking her concerns and reassuring her may be the difference between a traumatic event and one she remembers positively. All staff should have this as a priority and although the staff-member's conversation may not be having any impact on the mother, it is not considerate of her feelings at this time. Asking them politely to moderate their conversation (h) is a sensible approach. Rather than start chastising them in theatre which is likely to cause ructions in the team dynamic and worsen the atmosphere in the room, it would be wise to discuss afterwards with the line manager to see how the situation can be avoided in future (b).

65.
Eliminate the clearly wrong: d, f, h
These represent excessive first actions without actually dealing with the situation at the time
Best answers: a, c, e
Patient safety comes first (a), and it is important to check that other patients

have not come to harm (e). It is then important to address why the errors are happening in the first place (c), and offer your colleague support if appropriate. It is not your responsibility to apologise on their behalf (b). It may be necessary to complete an incident form (g), or involve seniors (d) at a later stage.

66.
Eliminate clearly wrong: a, d, g
Sedation should be a last line not first line option and putting yourself in danger achieves nothing either
Best answers: c, f, h

You should try to de-escalate the situation by talking to the patient and asking them to go to bed C. It is also advisable to familiarise yourself with the patient's case F. If conservative measures fail it may be necessary to medicate the patient and call security, but you should seek advice from a senior colleague before doing so H. Unless the nurse is seriously injured, you should deal with the on-going threat first. Never put yourself in harm's way, and when sedating a patient in such situations you should always choose oral medications before injections.

67.
Eliminate as clearly wrong: b, g, h
None of these address the matter in hand directly
Best answers: d, e, f
It is important that you quickly and discretely end the exchange between the doctor and nurse. Bring your colleague out of earshot of the patient and advise that he apologises to both other parties (e, f). The nurse might be struggling with their tasks and if you can help it will endear you to them (d). While incident forms are often used following this sort of altercation they are primarily for matters of patient safety. Informing the F1's consultant will be necessary if they are unwilling to resolve matters themselves.

68.
Best answers: c, d, g
Eliminate as clearly wrong: a, b, e
Although a patient has a right to confidentiality there are certain circumstances whereby confidentiality can be breached. In this instance, the decision of the patient to continue driving is not only putting his own life at risk, but also the life of others on the roads. In this situation, your duty to society overrides that of any individuals' confidentiality. With this in mind, the DVLA should be informed (C) so that they can take further and appropriate action to prevent the patient from driving. It would also be good practice to have a further discussion with the patient (G) to check that he fully realises the situation and better understand his reasons for continuing to drive or whether he previously misunderstood your instructions. Failing this, a discussion with the next of kin (D), who would already be aware of the driving limitation, would be prudent as they may be able to get through to the patient better.
Although writing a reflection in your ePortfolio (B), will help with your learning and professional progression, it is not useful in resolving the situation. Although

the GP may have a good rapport with the patient, asking them to have a discussion with the patient (H) is not good medical practice as you are the responsible clinician and you cannot guarantee this conversation will be had. At this stage calling the police (F) would not be appropriate and would lead to a large breakdown in trust and doctor-patient relationship, as would taking the keys from the patient (E), which is not your legal right. Ignoring the situation (A), is putting both the patient and other members of society at risk, and is therefore inappropriate.

69.
Best answers: b, g, h
Eliminate clearly wrong: a, c, d, e f
This question focuses on your ability to communicate in difficult circumstances. This lady is clearly terrified and needs some time and reassurance, both from you (h) and from family (b) if they are nearby and able to support her. You also need to communicate with your consultant early in the day (g) as if she refuses it has big implications for the theatre list and so it would be useful for them to know so that they can get another patient ready for theatre if they need to. Clearly signing an adult with incapacity form (h) is highly inappropriate for someone who has capacity and equally you cannot force someone to go to theatre who has capacity and is refusing. Leaving it up to your registrar (c) is unprofessional and if you reassure her before then the consent procedure is likely to be much smoother. Lastly referring her immediately to a nursing home is obviously wrong before she has had a chance at theatre, rehab and a chance to make a decision about her future need (d).

70.
Best answers: a, c, e
Eliminate clearly wrong: b, d, g, h
End of life care and planning is an important issue and one often skirted even by senior staff due to its difficult nature. Here it sounds like you have taken an appropriate decision in line with the patient and their family's wishes with your consultant's agreement. The best answers here as ever deal with the matter at hand while getting more information and help. Answer (a) may give more of an explanation why the consultant felt it was inappropriate including things you may have been unaware of. (a) goes hand in hand with (c, e) though as these give you senior backing and will be better received. It may be tempting to involve a registrar but this unfair on them and unlikely to have the same effect as involving the appropriate consultants. Likewise changing your practice or ignoring the email are also wrong and an incident report is quite vindictive. Gaining more information via your friend is tempting but is likely to be biased and may contain some conjecture so is less likely to be helpful.

Printed in Great
Britain
by Amazon